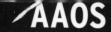
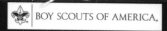 BOY SCOUTS OF AMERICA.

Wilderness First Aid
Field Guide

Alton L. Thygerson, EdD, EMT, FAW

Steven M. Thygerson, PhD, EMT, M

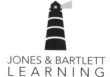

JONES & BARTLETT
LEARNING

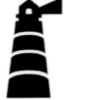

Jones and Bartlett Publishers
World Headquarters
Jones and Bartlett Publishers
40 Tall Pine Drive, Sudbury, MA 01776
978-443-5000
info@jbpub.com
www.ECSInstitute.org

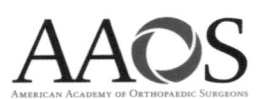

AMERICAN ACADEMY OF ORTHOPAEDIC SURGEONS

American Academy of Orthopaedic Surgeons
Editorial Credits
Chief Education Officer: Mark W. Wieting
Director, Department of Publications:
Marilyn L. Fox, PhD
Managing Editor: Barbara A. Scotese

Production Credits
Publisher, Public Safety: Kimberly Brophy
Associate Editor: Janet Morris
Production Editor: Karen Ferreira
Text and Cover Design: Anne Spencer
Manufacturing Buyer: Therese Connell
Composition: Shepherd, Inc.
Cover Photo: © Mellow Rapp/ShutterStock, Inc.
Printing and Binding: John P. Pow Company

ISBN-13: 978-1-4496-4123-8

The first aid procedures in this book are based on the most current recommendations of responsible medical sources. The American Academy of Orthopaedic Surgeons and the publisher, however, make no guarantee as to, and assume no responsibility for, the correctness, sufficiency, or completeness of such information or recommendations. Other or additional safety measures may be required under particular circumstances.

The content of this field guide exceeds the current Boy Scouts of America (BSA) Wilderness Curriculum. When training Boy Scouts using the BSA Wilderness Curriculum, sections of this guide will be omitted.

Additional credits appear on page 131, which constitutes a continuation of the copyright page.
6048

Printed in United States of America
15 14   10 9 8

Contents

Introduction   **1**

   Abbreviations/Mnemonics Used   **3**

   Signaling for Help   **3**

      Signaling Aircraft   *3*

      Other Signals   *4*

   Evacuation   **6**

      Guidelines for Helicopter Evacuation   *7*

      Guidelines for Ground Evacuation   *8*

   First Aid Kits   **9**

      Basic Survival Kit: The Bare Essentials   *13*

   Finding Out What Is Wrong   **14**

      Scene Survey   *14*

      Victim Assessment   *14*

A–Z of Injuries and Sudden Illnesses   **19**

   Abdominal Complaints   **19**

      Abdominal Pain   *19*

      Nausea and Vomiting   *20*

      Diarrhea   *21*

      Constipation   *22*

   Abdominal Injuries   **23**

Alcohol and Drug Emergencies   23

Alcohol Intoxication   23
Drugs   24

Allergic Reactions (Severe)   24

Altitude Illnesses   25

Acute Mountain Sickness (AMS)   25
High Altitude Pulmonary Edema (HAPE)   25
High Altitude Cerebral Edema (HACE)   25
Other Altitude-Related Illnesses   26

Arthropod Bites and Stings   27

Stinging Insects   29
Spider   30
Scorpion   31
Centipede   31
Tick   31
Chigger Mite   32
Mosquito   33
Fleas   33

Asthma   33

Bleeding and Wound Care   34

Wound Care   34
Infected Wound   36
Blood Under a Nail   37
Amputations   37
Animal Bites   39
Blisters   39

Fishhook Removal	41
Internal Bleeding	42
Bone, Joint, and Muscle Injuries	**43**
Broken Bones (Fractures)	43
Dislocated Joints: Shoulder, Kneecap, and Finger	45
Ankle Injuries	49
Knee Injuries	50
Splinting Guidelines	50
Muscle Injuries	52
Burns	**53**
Evacuation	55
Cardiac Arrest	**56**
CPR	56
CPR in Remote Locations	58
AED	60
Chest Injuries	**60**
Chest Pain	**61**
Choking	**62**
Diabetic Emergencies	**64**
Low Blood Sugar	65
High Blood Sugar	65
Eye Injuries	**66**
Female Health Problems	**68**
Vaginitis	68
Urinary Tract Infection	68

Contents

Vaginal Bleeding 69
Pregnancy Problems 69
Frostbite 69
Frostnip 71
Immersion Foot 72
Head Injuries 73
Scalp Wound 73
Skull Fracture 73
Brain Injury (Concussion) 74
Evacuation of Head-Injured Person 75
Heart Attack 76
Heat-Related Illnesses 76
Heatstroke 77
Heat Exhaustion 78
Heat Cramps 80
Heat Syncope 80
Heat Edema 81
Heat Rash (Prickly Heat) 81
Hypothermia 81
Mild Hypothermia 82
Severe Hypothermia 83
Lightning Injuries 85
Marine-Animal Injuries 86
Motion Sickness 87
Near-Drowning (Submersion) 88

Nose Injuries	89
Plant-Related Problems	90
Plant-Induced Dermatitis: Poison Ivy, Poison Oak, and Poison Sumac	*90*
Cactus Spines	*93*
Stinging Nettle	*94*
Swallowed (Ingested) Poisonous Plant	*94*
Seizures	96
Shock	97
Snake and Other Reptile Bites	98
Spinal Cord Injury	101
Stroke (Brain Attack)	104
Tooth Injuries	105
Wild Animal Attacks	107
Prevention	**108**
Altitude Illness	108
Avalanche Burial	109
Bear Attack	110
Blisters	113
Cold-Related Emergencies	114
Conserve, Share, and Create Warmth	*116*
Clothing	*117*

Dehydration   118
  How Much Fluid to Drink?   *118*
Drowning   119
Heat Stress   120
Insect Stings (Bees, Wasps, Hornets,
    and Yellow Jackets)   122
Lightning Strike   123
Mosquito Bites   125
Mountain Lion Attack   125
Poisonous Plant Dermatitis   126
Snakebite   127
Tick Bite   127
Waterborne Diseases   129
  Boiling   *129*
  Chemicals   *130*
  Special Filters   *130*

Photo Credits   **131**

Introduction

Everyone should be prepared for injuries and medical problems when in situations (e.g., the wilderness) in which professional medical care is not readily available. The Wilderness Medical Society defines "wilderness" as being more than 1 hour away from definitive medical care. Thus, you may be in a wilderness environment without realizing it. Some activities, places, and events that can cause you to be in a wilderness situation include the following:

- Personal recreation (e.g., campers, hikers, hunters, rafters, birders, skiers, and climbers)
- Remote occupations (e.g., farmers, foresters, linesmen, and ranchers)
- Remote residences (e.g., small communities, farms, ranches, and vacation homes)
- Remote locations (e.g., remote parts of North America and developing countries)
- Disasters (e.g., winter storms, hurricanes, earthquakes, tornadoes, and floods)

Those far from medical help may be confronted with the following:

- Delayed or prolonged evacuation because of bad weather, a difficult location, or a lack of transportation or communication

- Adverse conditions (e.g., heat, cold, rain, snow, and altitude)
- Limited first aid supplies and equipment (e.g., restricted to portable and/or improvisation)
- Injuries and illnesses not seen in urban areas (e.g., altitude illness, frostbite, and wild animal attacks)
- The need for advanced care (e.g., reducing some dislocations and wound care)
- The need to make difficult decisions (e.g., CPR and evacuation)

The purpose of this guide is to prepare you for victim assessment and care in all of these situations. It contains current emergency care recommendations from the Wilderness Medical Society's *Practice Guidelines for Wilderness Emergency Care,* the Wilderness Medical Society and American Academy of Orthopaedic Surgeon's book *Wilderness First Aid: Emergency Care for Remote Locations,* protocols from the National Association of EMS Physicians and the State of Alaska Cold Injuries Guidelines, and current medical literature.

These guidelines should not be considered final, as they will be constantly updated to reflect current standards of care. The authors and publisher will not be held responsible, nor assume liability, in respect to the accuracy or implementation of the information or treatment guidelines in this guide.

Abbreviations/Mnemonics Used

AVPU = alert and aware, responds to voice, responds to pain, unresponsive

CPR = cardiopulmonary resuscitation

DOTS = deformity, open wounds, tenderness, swelling

SAMPLE = symptoms (known as the chief complaint), allergies, medications, past pertinent illnesses, last fluid/food, previous events

RICE = rest, ice, compression, elevation

Signaling for Help

Many emergency conditions require a search for people in distress. Under such circumstances, it is always better if those being sought know how to make their presence and location conspicuous.

Signaling Aircraft

The key to any ground signal is that very few straight lines or right angles exist in nature. Remember that things appear a lot smaller when viewed from the air, and thus, bigger is almost always better. For ground signals, make a large V for immediate assistance or an X if medical assistance is needed. Make the lines of these signals as large as you can.

Construct your signal using a ratio of six to one (e.g., a **V** with sides 12 × 2 feet). Contrast is another key to ground signals. Examples of materials to use include toilet paper, strips of plastic tarp, strips of tent material, tree branches, logs, and light-colored rocks. In snow, on the open ground, or on a beach, signals may be tramped or dug into the surface using shadows to make the signals stand out.

Other Signals

A series of three signals in quick succession indicates "help." Examples include three shouts, three shots, three blasts from a whistle, and three flashes from a light.

Use smoke by day and bright flame by night if other signaling devices are not available. Add engine oil, rags soaked in oil, or pieces of rubber to your fire to make black smoke (best against light background). Add green leaves, moss, or a little water to send up billows of white smoke (best against dark background). If tending a fire while waiting for help, keep plenty of fuel at hand. Throw it on the fire the moment an aircraft is heard—it takes time for smoke to form and rise.

A mirror is an effective means of sending a distress signal. On hazy days, an aircraft can see the flash of a mirror before survivors can see the aircraft; it is wise to flash the mirror in the direction of a plane when you hear it, even if you cannot see it. Mirror flashes have been spotted by rescue aircraft more than 20 miles away.

To use a mirror, follow this procedure:

1. Hold the mirror up to the sun with one hand, and stretch your other hand in front of you, holding up a finger or thumb so that it blots out the view of your target.
2. Hit your extended finger or thumb with a reflection of the sun from the mirror.
3. Repeatedly flick the spot of light from the mirror across the finger or thumb and the aircraft.
4. Try to hit the aircraft or rescuers with a flash as much as possible. Do not attempt to do a series of three flashes—it is too difficult. Figure 1

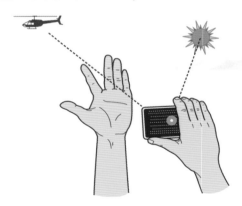

Figure 1

[Evacuation*]

A victim's health or survival may depend on moving them to medical care. Determining the best method (e.g., helicopter versus carrying versus walking) must be based on several factors:

- Severity of the illness or injury
- Rescue and medical skill of rescuers
- Physical and psychological condition of rescuers and victim
- Availability of equipment and aid for the rescue
- Amount of time—determined by distance, terrain, weather, and other conditions—that it would take to evacuate the victim
- Cost

It is usually best to postpone further travel and/or initiate evacuation from the wilderness for any person who has the following:

- Worsening symptoms, such as:
  - Altered mental status
  - Unrelieved vomiting or diarrhea
  - An inability to tolerate drinking fluids
  - Return of unresponsiveness after a head injury

---

* This is adapted from and based on the Wilderness Medical Society *Practice Guidelines for Wilderness Emergency Care.*

- Debilitating pain
- Inability to travel at a reasonable pace because of a medical problem
- Sustained abdominal pain
- Passage of blood by mouth or rectum (not from an obviously minor source)
- Serious high-altitude illness signs and symptoms
- Infections that worsen despite appropriate treatment
- Chest pain that is not clearly musculoskeletal in origin
- Development of a dysfunctional psychological status that impairs the safety of the person or group
- Large or severe wounds or a wound with complications (e.g., open fracture, deformed fracture, a suspected spinal injury, a fracture or dislocation impairing circulation to arm or leg)

Guidelines for Helicopter Evacuation

Helicopters can reduce the time to medical care. Evacuate by helicopter only if the following applies:
- The victim's life will be saved.
- The victim will have a significantly better chance for full recovery.
- The pilot believes conditions are safe enough for helicopter evacuation.
- Ground evacuation would be dangerous or prolonged or has a deficient number of rescuers.

Helicopter Safety Rules

The main hazards are the main rotor blades and the tail rotor (appears nearly invisible during operation).

- Approach the helicopter from the front where the pilot can see you.
- Never walk downhill to approach the helicopter. Never walk uphill when exiting a helicopter.
- Board only when the pilot approves.
- Secure all loose clothing and equipment.
- Never chase an item that has blown away. Wait for the helicopter to land.
- Protect eyes from the rotor downwash. If blinded by debris, stop and kneel. Someone will come to help.
- Do not stand in the landing zone, and clear debris from the landing zone before the helicopter's arrival.

Guidelines for Ground Evacuation

If the victim is walking out, at least two people should accompany him or her. If the victim is unable to continue, one person can stay with the victim while the other goes for help.

If the victim is being carried out:

- Send someone to notify authorities that help is needed.
- At least four, preferably six, bearers should carry the stretcher (litter) at all times.

- Over rough terrain, eight carriers (six over smooth trail) should carry the litter for 15 minutes and then rest or rotate with other carriers.

Even when rescue help is requested (e.g., cell phone), a detailed written note describing the situation and victim's condition should be completed. When without a cell phone, one or two members of the party can carry out a written request for help.

First Aid Kits

Most injuries and sudden illnesses do not require medical care. For all remote locations, it is a good idea to have useful supplies for emergencies.

A first aid kit's supplies should be customized to include those items that are likely to be used on a regular basis. The list includes nonprescription (over-the-counter) medications. Some medications lose their potency over time, especially after they have been opened; check expiration dates twice a year. Keep all medicines out of the reach of children. Read and follow all directions for proper medication use. The following list contains useful first aid kit items. Change the list to meet the needs of situations that you are likely to encounter.

Item	Use
Alcohol hand sanitizer gel (small bottle)	Cleans hands and the area around the wound (not inside wound)
Antibiotic ointment (Polysporin, Neosporin, bacitracin, triple-antibiotic ointment)	Prevents skin infections that are associated with shallow wounds and makes nonstick dressings
Aloe vera gel (100% gel)	Apply to skin for sunburn or superficial frostbite.
Moleskin/molefoam	Apply over "hot spots" before blister formation. Several layers cut into a "doughnut" shape are useful for painful blisters.
Irrigation syringe (10 cc or 20 cc)	Provides pressure irrigation of wounds
Bandage strips (various sizes, also known as Band-Aids)	Covers minor wounds
Sterile gauze pads (2" x 2" and 4" x 4", individually wrapped)	Covers wounds
Nonsticking pads	Covers burns, blisters, and scrapes
Self-adhering roller bandage (2" to 4" wide; Kerlix, Kling)	Holds dressings
Sterile trauma pad (5" x 9", 8" x 10")	Covers large wounds
Elastic bandage (4" wide; Ace wrap)	Provides compression to reduce the swelling of joint injuries
Adhesive tape—various types available (e.g., athletic tape, hypoallergenic tape, waterproof tape)	Secures dressings and splints
Duct tape (very small roll)	Covers skin "hot spots" before a blister forms, holds a dressing or splint, and has many other uses
Safety pins (2" long)	Creates sling from shirttail or sleeve, secure dressings, and drain blisters

(continued)

Item	Use
Pain and anti-inflammatory medication: For children, use acetaminophen (Tylenol); for adults, use aspirin or ibuprofen (Advil, Motrin).	Treats pain, fever, and swelling. Give only acetaminophen for children. Acetaminophen does not reduce swelling.
Decongestant tablets (e.g., Sudafed) Decongestant spray (e.g., Afrin, Neo-Synephrine)	Relieves nasal and upper respiratory congestion of viral "colds," allergies, and sinus infections Spray can be helpful in controlling nosebleeds.
Antihistamine (e.g., Benadryl)	Relieves allergy symptoms and treats poison ivy or oak itching and rash. It reduces nausea and motion sickness, causes drowsiness, and induces sleep.
Antibiotic ointment (e.g., Neosporin, Bacitracin, Polysporin)	Treats shallow wounds
Hydrocortisone cream, 1%	Soothes inflammation associated with insect bites and stings, poison ivy and oak, and other allergic skin rashes. It may be too weak for some conditions.
Calamine lotion (tends to be in large bottles and thus may not be practical to carry)	Anti-itch and drying agent for poison ivy or oak and skin rashes
Commercial sport drink packets (e.g., Gatorade)	Treats heat stress, dehydration, and "water intoxication" when too much water has been consumed and sodium has been depleted from body.
Sunscreen lotion (with sun protection factor of at least 15)	Prevents sunburn and windburn

(continued)

Item	Use
Lip balm (with sun protection factor of 15)	Prevents sunburn and chapping of lips and soothes cold sores
Insect repellent with DEET (< 30%)	Repels insects. For children, use no more than 10% DEET. Permethrin on clothes repels ticks.
Antacids tablets (e.g., Tums and Rolaids)	Treats heartburn and acid indigestion
Antidiarrheal tablets (e.g., Pepto-Bismol and Imodium A-D)	Treats diarrhea
Anticonstipation (e.g., Metamucil)	Treats constipation
Scissors (various types are available)	Cut dressings, bandages, and clothing
Tweezers (angled tip)	Removes splinters and ticks
Thermometer, digital (if available, 75° F to 105° F)	Measures fever
SAM splint	Stabilizes broken bones and dislocations
Medical exam gloves	Protects against potentially infected blood and body fluids
Mouth-to-barrier device	Protects against potential infection during rescue breathing/CPR.
Emergency blanket (e.g., state highway department trash bags; household polyethylene trash bags; "space" blanket made of Mylar, although may tear in wind)	Protects against body heat loss and weather (wind, rain, and snow)
Small notebook/pencil	Records information
Small first aid manual	Quick reference during an emergency and is used for learning first aid procedures

Basic Survival Kit: The Bare Essentials

Carry this kit whenever you are in remote areas.

Minimal Items	Purpose
One or two large, heavy duty plastic bags (similar to state highway department trash bags), household polyethylene trash bags, or emergency blanket ("space blanket") made of mylar—may tear in wind	Protection against weather (wind, rain, snow). Wear one trash bag by cutting hole in bottom of bag for head to fit through; use the second bag to cover legs.
Whistle*	Signal for help.
Signal mirror**	Signal for help.
Metal match with striker (magnesium)	Start a fire.
Waterproof match case containing windproof/waterproof matches	Start a fire.
Waterproof match case or empty film canister containing several cotton balls smeared with Vaseline	Petroleum jelly is flammable. Make tinder using cotton balls smeared with petroleum jelly. When using, open the cotton ball to catch sparks from metal match.
Knife (multitool) and/or wire blade survival saw	Used for cutting
Food***	Provides calories and a psychological boost

* Whistle: A whistle is far superior to shouting. The whistle will carry for 0.5 to 2.0 miles or more in the wilderness, whereas your voice may only carry a few hundred yards. You will be able to signal for longer periods of time. Give three blasts in succession, repeated at intervals, to get attention. New high-tech whistles such as the "Storm" (from ALL-Weather Safety Whistle Co.) and the "Fox 40" (from Fox 40 International) and the smaller, more compact versions of these super whistles, the "WindStorm" and the "Mini-Fox 40," are much louder than police or referee whistles.

** Signal mirror: A mirror of 4 × 5 inches (standard U.S. Coast Guard size) or 3 × 5 inches is ideal, but the smaller 2 × 3 inch size also works well. Specially made glass and plastic signal mirrors are available. If you do not have a mirror, improvise using any piece of metal (polish it with fine sand or dirt), foil, or any shiny object. A mirror works even on overcast days and with moonlight, although with reduced range.
*** Food: Good items to carry include energy bars, candy bars, hard candy (e.g., lemon drops), powdered chocolate, dehydrated soup, or MREs (the U.S. military surplus meals-ready-to-eat). Discard any with soon-to-lapse expiration dates.

Finding Out What Is Wrong

Scene Survey

In most cases:

1. Take charge of the situation. If someone is already in charge, ask whether you can help. If you suspect head/spinal injuries, tell the victim not to move.
2. Shout for help to attract nearby bystanders (see the Signaling for Help section).
3. Scan for hazards. If the scene is unsafe, make it safe. If unable to do so, do not enter.
4. Determine the number of victims.
5. Determine the mechanism of injury (cause of injury) for each victim to help identify what is wrong.
6. Identify yourself as a first aid provider. Offer to help, and obtain consent from the victim.

Victim Assessment

Primary Check

The initial victim assessment identifies immediate life-threatening conditions involving the airway and breathing—

in which complications can result in death if not attended to within minutes (refer to the Cardiac Arrest section for the procedures). After the initial assessment, a physical exam and SAMPLE history can reveal other problems needing first aid.

Secondary Check

Perform a secondary check by looking and feeling for DOTS:

D = **D**eformity
O = **O**pen wounds
T = **T**enderness
S = **S**welling

Start at the head and end at the feet. Most victims will not need a complete head-to-toe exam. Instead, they will be able to tell you their main complaint, and you can direct your attention to that area.

SAMPLE History

Description	Sample Questions
S = **S**ymptoms	"What is wrong?" (known as the chief complaint)
A = **A**llergies	"Are you allergic to anything?"
M = **M**edications	"Are you taking any medications? What are they for?"
P = **P**ast medical history	"Have you had this problem before? Do you have other medical problems?" *(continued)*

Description	Sample Questions
L = **L**ast oral intake	"When did you last eat or drink anything? What was it?"
E = **E**vent leading up to the illness or injury	Injury: "How did you get hurt?" Illness: "What led to this problem?"

Putting It All Together: Victim Assessment Sequence

1. Determine the responsiveness (most victims are responsive).
2. Perform an initial assessment (most victims will not have life-threatening conditions).
3. Determine whether the victim is injured or ill.

Sequence of Victim Assessment

	Injured Victim			Suddenly Ill Victim	
		Responsive			
Unresponsive	**With Significant COI**	**Without Significant COI**	**Unresponsive**	**Responsive**	
· Primary check · Secondary check using the DOS parts of DOTS · Sample history from others	· Primary check · Secondary check using DOTS · SAMPLE history	· Primary check · Examine chief complaint using DOTS · SAMPLE history	· Primary check · Secondary check using the DOS parts of DOTS · SAMPLE history from others	· Primary check · SAMPLE history · Examine chief complaint	

COI = cause of injury; also known as mechanism of injury. DOTS = deformity, open wounds, tenderness, swelling. SAMPLE = symptoms, allergies, medications, pertinent history, last oral intake, and events leading up to the illness or injury.

Significant Causes of Injury (COI)

- Falls >3× victim's height
- Vehicles (sport utility vehicles [SUVs], trucks, cars, motorcycles, bicycles, all-terrain vehicles [ATVs], snowmobiles) involving ejection, rollovers, high-speeds
- Unresponsive or altered mental status (V, P, or U on AVPU scale)
- Penetrations (head, chest, ABD)

Medical Identification Tags

A medical alert tag (e.g., bracelet, necklace) contains the wearer's medical problem(s) and a 24-hour telephone number. The tag can sometimes help identify what is wrong with the victim.

How Responsive? The AVPU Scale

A = **A**lert and aware (eyes open; can answer questions clearly; knows name, place, and day of week)
V = Responds to **V**oice (might not know name, place, and day of week)
P = Responds to **P**ain (eyes do not open; no response to questions; responds to pinching of muscle above collarbone)
U = **U**nresponsive (eyes do not open, no response to pinching of muscle above collarbone)

Avoid negative statements that may add to victim's distress, fear, and pain. Use simple words to create confidence, comfort, and cooperation.

1. Your first words to a victim are very important.
2. Do not ask unnecessary questions (e.g., "What did you do?") unless it aids treatment or satisfies the victim's need to talk.
3. Make no negative value judgments.
4. Link a suggestion that you want the injured person to accept with a statement he or she cannot deny (e.g., "that leg is probably hurting, but we'll soon make you comfortable").
5. Tears and/or laughter can be normal—let the injured person know this if such responses seem to make him or her feel embarrassed or guilty.
6. Stress the positive (e.g., instead of "you will not have any pain," say "you will feel better").
7. Do not deny the obvious (e.g., instead of saying that "there is nothing wrong," say that "you've had quite a fall and probably don't feel too good, but we're going to look after you; you'll soon be feeling better").

[Abdominal Complaints]

Abdominal Pain

There are many possible causes of abdominal pain, some not so serious and some life threatening. Some can be serious enough to require immediate evacuation for medical care. Illnesses affecting the abdomen have two things in common: they are very painful, and even skilled physicians may have trouble pinpointing an exact cause. It is impractical for a first aid provider to distinguish among the many causes of abdominal pain because first aid will usually be similar regardless of the cause.

What to Do

1. Give water or clear fluids such as sports drinks, clear soups, or apple juice (no alcohol or caffeine). Have victim slowly sip the fluids. Avoid solid foods. Later give clear soups and bland foods (e.g., toast, oatmeal).
2. Give victim an antacid (e.g., Tums, Rolaids, Pepto-Bismol). If these fail, try a medication that helps stop stomach acid secretion (e.g., Tagamet and Pepcid AC). If these fail, seek medical advice.
3. If practical, place a hot-water bottle against the victim's abdomen, or have the victim soak in a warm bath.

4. Be prepared for vomiting.
5. Keep the victim lying down with knees bent. Evacuate to medical help if any of these apply:
   - Pain is constant for more than 6 hours.
   - The victim is unable to eat or drink fluids.
   - The victim is or may be pregnant.
   - Significant recent abdominal injury exists.
   - The abdomen is rigid and painful.
   - After pressing your fingers on victim's abdomen and suddenly releasing it, more pain occurs.
   - There is bloody, blood-stained, or black stool.
   - The victim has a high fever.
   - Pain began around the navel (belly button) and later moved to the lower right abdomen.

Nausea and Vomiting

Vomiting and nausea often occur with conditions such as acute mountain sickness, motion sickness, brain injury, intestinal viruses, eating or drinking too much, and being emotionally upset.

What to Do

1. Give water or clear fluids such as sports drinks, clear soups, and apple juice (no alcohol or caffeine). Have victim slowly sip the fluids. Avoid solid foods. Later give clear soups and bland foods (e.g., toast, crackers, and oatmeal).
2. Rest and avoid exertion until the victim is able to eat solid foods easily.

3. Be prepared for vomiting.
4. Evacuate to medical help if any of these apply:
   - Blood or brown, grainy material appears in vomit.
   - Constant abdominal pain exists.
   - Victim faints when standing.
   - Victim is unable to keep fluids down for more than 24 hours.
   - Vomiting follows a recent head injury.

Diarrhea

Diarrhea is the frequent (usually more than four times a day) passage of loose, watery, or unformed stools. Some experts say to let diarrhea run its course because bacteria or parasites are expelled and are not trapped in the intestines.

What to Do

1. Give water or clear fluids such as sports drinks, clear soups, or apple juice (no alcohol or caffeine). Have the victim slowly sip the fluids. Avoid solid foods. Later give clear soups and bland foods (e.g., toast, crackers, oatmeal).
2. Give Pepto-Bismol (follow the label directions). It can turn the stool and tongue black. Those who are sensitive to aspirin should not use it. If the victim must be in control of his or her stools, Imodium A-D can reduce the movement of food through the intestines.

3. Evacuate to medical help if any of these apply:
   - Blood in stools that may appear black (keep in mind that Pepto-Bismol can cause black stools)
   - No improvement after 24 hours
   - Fever
   - Severe, constant abdominal pain
   - Severe dehydration

Constipation

Constipation is the passage of hard, dry stools occurring fewer than three times a week.

What to Do
1. Make sure the victim drinks plenty of fluids (8 to 10 eight-ounce cups daily).
2. Have the victim eat fiber (fresh or dried fruits, vegetables, or bran). Over-the-counter fiber products (e.g., Metamucil or Citrucel) can be used (follow label directions). *Do not* give a laxative.
3. Encourage the victim to remain active.
4. If no improvement occurs, try milk of magnesia or caffeine.
5. Evacuate to medical help if any of these apply:
   - Severe abdominal pain
   - Visibly swollen abdomen accompanied by pain
   - Fever
   - Vomiting

[Abdominal Injuries]

What to Look For	What to Do
Penetrating object	**DO NOT** remove a penetrating object. Stabilize the object against movement. **DO NOT** give the victim anything to eat or drink. Evacuate to medical help.
Protruding organs	**DO NOT** try to reinsert protruding organs back into the abdomen. **DO NOT** touch organs. Cover them with a moist, clean dressing. **DO NOT** give the victim anything to eat or drink. Evacuate to medical help.
Hard blow to abdomen	Roll the victim on one side in case of vomiting. **DO NOT** give the victim anything to eat or drink. Evacuate to medical help.

[Alcohol and Drug Emergencies]

Alcohol Intoxication

What to Look For	What to Do
· Odor of alcohol · Unsteady, staggering walking · Slurred speech and unable to carry on a conversation · Nausea and vomiting · Flushed face	1. Monitor breathing. 2. Check for injuries. 3. Keep in the recovery position.

A

Drugs

Drugs are classified according to their effects on the user.

What to Look For	What to Do
• **Uppers** stimulate the central nervous system. Examples are amphetamines and cocaine. • **Downers** depress the central nervous system. Examples are barbiturates, tranquilizers, marijuana, and narcotics. • **Hallucinogens** alter the senses (e.g., vision). Examples are LSD, mescaline, peyote, and PCP (angel dust). Marijuana also has some hallucinogenic capabilities. • **Volatile chemicals** usually are inhaled and can seriously damage many body organs. Examples are paint solvents, gasoline, and spray paint.	1. Monitor breathing. 2. Check for injuries. 3. Keep in recovery position. 4. Seek medical help.

Warning
- *Do not* let an intoxicated or drugged person sleep on his or her back.
- *Do not* leave an intoxicated or drugged person alone.
- *Do not* try to handle a violent person by yourself—find a safe place, and call law enforcement officials.

Allergic Reactions (Severe)

Reactions to medications, food and food additives, insect stings, and plant pollen can be life threatening (called anaphylaxis).

What to Look For	What to Do
• Warm feeling followed by intense itching • Skin flushes; face may swell • Sneezing, coughing, wheezing • Shortness of breath • Tightness and swelling in the throat • Tightness in the chest • Increased pulse • Swelling of tongue, mouth, nose • Blueness around lips and mouth • Dizziness • Nausea and vomiting	1. Monitor breathing. 2. Seek medical help as soon as possible. 3. If the victim has his or her own physician-prescribed epinephrine, help the victim use it. 4. Give antihistamine (Benadryl)—it is not life saving because it takes too long to work, but can prevent further reactions.

[Altitude Illnesses]

Going above 8,000 feet can produce one of several types of altitude sickness because of a lack of oxygen and decreased barometric pressure in the blood and tissues. Figure 2

Acute Mountain Sickness (AMS)	High-Altitude Pulmonary Edema (HAPE)	High-Altitude Cerebral Edema (HACE)
Above 8,000 feet for 1 to 2 days: • Headache, usually throbbing	Above 10,000 feet for 3 to 4 days (can be life threatening): • Shortness of breath	Above 12,000 feet for 4 to 7 days (can be life threatening): • Severe headache *(continued)*

Acute Mountain Sickness (AMS)	High-Altitude Pulmonary Edema (HAPE)	High-Altitude Cerebral Edema (HACE)
· Sleep disturbance · Fatigue · Shortness of breath · Dizziness · Loss of appetite · Vomiting	· Dry cough · Mild chest pain · Weakness · Insomnia · Rapid pulse · Crackling or gurgling	· Vomiting · Cannot walk straight · Unresponsive
What to Do 1. Stop ascending or descend. 2. Drink fluids. 3. Rest. 4. Take pain medication. 5. A doctor prescribed medication can prevent this.	**What to Do** 1. It is the same as for AMS. 2. Descend immediately at least 2,000 feet. 3. Evacuate immediately to medical help.	**What to Do** 1. It is the same as for AMS. 2. Descend immediately 4,000 feet. 3. Evacuate as soon as possible to medical help.

Other Altitude-Related Illnesses

Pharyngitis and Bronchitis

Because of dry air, a sore throat and coughing may develop. The victim should drink fluids, have antibiotic ointment applied in the nose, and suck hard candy or throat lozenges. For dry coughing, give a cough medicine (e.g., Robitussin DM).

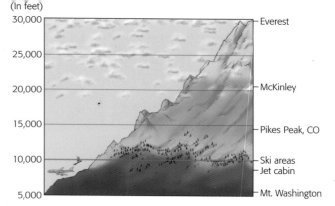

(In feet)

- 30,000 — Everest
- 25,000
- 20,000 — McKinley
- 15,000 — Pikes Peak, CO
- 10,000 — Ski areas / Jet cabin
- 5,000 — Mt. Washington

Figure 2

Peripheral Edema

Swelling of hands, ankles, and/or face (around eyes) may appear at higher altitudes. If possible, raise the victim's arms and/or legs. After descending or with acclimatization to higher altitudes, the swelling diminishes. Descend if signs of more serious altitude illnesses appear.

Arthropod Bites and Stings

Arthropods—including scorpions, spiders, centipedes, and ticks—are invertebrates with jointed legs and segmented bodies. Stinging insects cause more deaths than do snakes. Figures 3-6

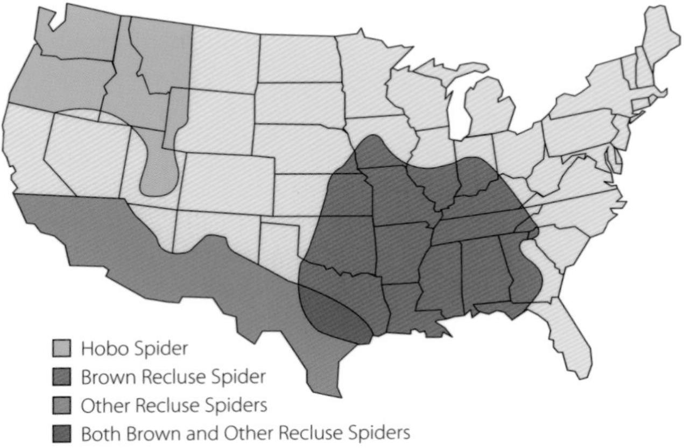

Arthropod Bites and Stings

[Map of United States]

☐ Hobo Spider
☐ Brown Recluse Spider
☐ Other Recluse Spiders
☐ Both Brown and Other Recluse Spiders

Figure 3

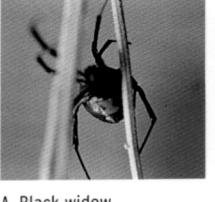

A. Black widow

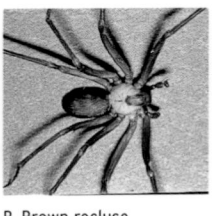

B. Brown recluse

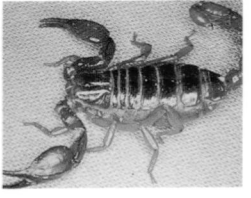

C. Scorpion

Figure 4

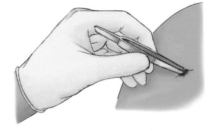

Figure 5

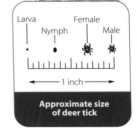

Larva
Nymph
Female
Male

← 1 inch →

Approximate size of deer tick

Figure 6

Arthropod	What to Look For	What to Do
Stinging insects · Honeybee · Bumblebee · Hornet · Yellow jacket · Wasp · Fire ants Those who have had a previous severe reaction should wear a medical-alert ID tag and carry a physician-prescribed epinephrine kit.	· Usual reactions: instant pain, redness, itching. · Worrisome reactions: hives, lips/tongue swell, "tickle" in throat, and wheezing. · Life-threatening reactions: blue/gray skin color, seizures, unresponsiveness, and inability to breathe because of swollen vocal cords. · About 60% to 80% of anaphylactic deaths are caused by victim's inability to breathe because of swollen airway passages.	1. Look for a stinger, and if found, remove it as soon as possible using any removal method (e.g., brush it away with your hand, scrape it with a fingernail or a knife blade). Do not use tweezers. Only bees leave their stinger embedded. 2. Wash with soap and water. 3. Apply ice pack. Baking soda paste may help except for wasp stings. 4. Give pain medication. Apply hydrocortisone (1%), and give antihistamine. *(continued)*

Arthropod Bites and Stings

Widow spider bites Best known as the black widow, but term "black widow" is inaccurate because only three of the five species of widow spiders are black, the others being brown and gray. Only adult females bite. They have a shiny, black abdomen with a red or yellow spot that is often in shape of hourglass, or white spots or bands on the abdomen.	• May feel sharp pinprick with dull, numbing pain developing • Two small fang marks seen as tiny red spots • Severe abdominal pain (bites on arm can produce severe chest pain, thus mimicking a heart attack) • Headache, chills, fever, heavy sweating, nausea, and vomiting Most victims never see the spider.	1. Clean with soap and water. 2. Apply an ice pack. 3. Give pain medication. 4. Evacuate to medical help.
Fiddle-back spider bites Also known as brown recluse spider, violin, and brown spiders.	• Mild to severe pain occurs within 2 to 8 hours. • A blister develops later, becomes red, and bursts. It takes a "bull's-eye" appearance. • Nausea, vomiting, headache, and fever	Same as for black widow spider. If wound becomes infected, apply antibiotic ointment under sterile dressing.
Hobo spider bites Also known as the aggressive house spider.	Same as for fiddle-back spiders.	Same as for fiddle-back spiders.

(continued)

Tarantula spider bites They bite only when vigorously provoked or roughly handled. They can flick their hairs onto a person's skin.	• Pain varies from mild to severe throbbing lasting up to 1 hour.	Same as for black widow spider. For hairs in the skin, wash with soap and water; apply hydrocortisone cream, and give antihistamine.
Scorpion stings In the United States, only the Bark Scorpion found in Arizona is potentially deadly—it is active from May through August.	• Burning pain • Numbness or tingling occurs later.	1. Monitor breathing. 2. Wash with soap and water. 3. Apply ice pack. 4. Give pain medication. 5. Apply dressing. 6. Evacuate to medical help for severe reactions.
Centipede bites Do not confuse with millipedes, which cannot inject venom but can irritate the skin.	• Burning pain • Inflammation • Mild swelling of lymph nodes	1. Wash with soap and water. 2. Apply ice pack. 3. Give pain medication. 4. Evacuate to medical help for severe reactions.
Embedded tick Most ticks are harmless, but can carry diseases. If it is carrying a disease, the longer it stays embedded, the greater the chance of the disease being transmitted.	• No pain initially exists, and it can go unnoticed for days without detection. • The bite varies from a small bump to extensive swelling and ulcer. • May cause fever, chills, and rash	Remove the tick: 1. Use tweezers or a specialized tick-removal tool to grasp tick close to skin and lift up to "tent" skin surface. Hold until tick lets go, or after about 1 minute, pull tick away from skin—**DO NOT** jerk or *(continued)*

twist tick. The remaining mouth parts do not transmit disease and will usually be expelled later.

2. Wash with soap and water.

3. Disinfect with rubbing alcohol.

4. Apply ice pack.

5. Check for rash for 1 month. If a rash appears, seek medical help.

Cautions:

- **DO NOT** use fingernail polish.
- **DO NOT** use rubbing alcohol.
- **DO NOT** use hot extinguished match head.
- **DO NOT** apply petroleum jelly.
- **DO NOT** apply gasoline.

Chigger mite bites
Bites can number in the 100s.

- Severe itching occurs after several hours.
- Small red welts appear.
- Skin infection can result.

1. Wash with soap and water and rinse several times.

2. Apply hydrocortisone (1%) ointment or calamine lotion.

3. Give antihistamine.

Effectiveness of applying clear nail polish is questionable.

(continued)

Mosquito bites Human breath (contains carbon dioxide) and sweat attract mosquitoes.	• Itching • Mild swelling	1. Wash with soap and water. 2. Apply hydrocortisone (1%) ointment. 3. Apply an ice pack. 4. Give an antihistamine.
Fleas	• Itching Multiple bites—termed "breakfast, lunch, and dinner"—are common.	1. Apply an ice pack. 2. Apply hydrocortisone (1%) ointment. 3. Give an antihistamine.

[Asthma]

Asthma is a respiratory illness with repeated attacks of shortness of breath, often with wheezing and coughing. Between the attacks the person has no trouble breathing. Asthma varies from one person to another, with symptoms ranging from mild to severe, and can be life threatening.

What to Look For	What to Do
• Coughing • Whistling noise during breathing • Bluish skin color • Inability to speak in complete sentences without stopping to breathe • Fast breathing • Victim sitting upright trying to breathe	1. Place the victim in an upright sitting position, leaning slightly forward. 2. Monitor breathing. 3. Help the victim take asthma medication. 4. If the victim does not respond well to inhaled medication or is having a severe attack, seek medical help. *Caution:* **DO NOT** wait too long to get medical help for a severe asthma attack.

[**Bleeding and Wound Care**]

Wound Care

1. Expose the bleeding wound.
2. Protect yourself against disease by wearing disposable medical exam gloves. If medical exam gloves are unavailable, use waterproof material, extra dressings, or clean cloths, or the victim can apply pressure with his or her own hand. Figure 7
3. Stop the bleeding by placing a sterile gauze pad or clean cloth over the wound and pressing directly over

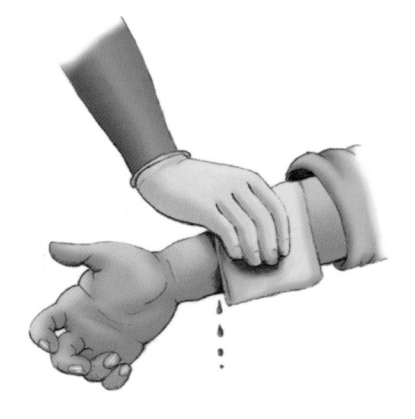

Figure 7

the wound. If bleeding does not stop in 10 minutes, press harder over a wider area for another 10 minutes. For a gaping wound, pack the wound with sterile dressing.

4. Clean the wound (this may restart bleeding):
   a. For a shallow wound:
      - Wash inside and around wound with soap and water.
      - Flush the inside of the wound with pressurized water that is clean enough to drink. This means water from a faucet or an irrigation syringe (10 or 20 cc). If using an irrigation syringe, flush 0.75 to 1 cup of water through the wound. Squeezing a plastic bag with a small hole may be helpful. Pouring, soaking, or using a bulb syringe does not provide enough pressure to be effective but may be all that is available.
      - Cover it with a thin layer of an over-the-counter antibiotic ointment (e.g., Neosporin or Poly-sporin). *Do not* use merthiolate, mercurochrome, or hydrogen peroxide.
   b. For a wound with a high risk for infection (e.g., animal bite, very dirty or ragged wound, puncture wound), clean the best you can. Evacuate to medical help as soon as possible.

5. Cover shallow and high-risk wounds with a sterile dressing. *Do not* close the wound with tape.
6. Evacuate to medical help to:
   - Clean wounds at high risk for infection.
   - Close wide and gaping open wounds or if an underlying structure (e.g., tendon, nerve) is injured.
   - Receive a possible tetanus booster.

When possible, scrub hands vigorously with soap and water before and after giving help. If water is unavailable, use an alcohol hand sanitizing gel.

Infected Wound

Any wound, large or small, can become infected. Proper cleaning can help prevent infections.

What to Look For	What to Do
• Swelling and redness around wound • Feels warmer than surrounding area • Throbbing pain • Pus discharge • Fever • Swelling of lymph nodes • One or more red streaks leading from the wound toward the heart, as this is a serious sign that the infection is spreading	1. Soak the wound in warm water, or apply warm, wet packs over the infected wound. 2. Apply an antibiotic ointment. 3. Change the dressings daily. 4. Give pain medication. 5. Evacuate to medical help.

Blood Under a Nail

What to Look For	What to Do
A fingernail or toenail has been crushed or smashed and has unbearable pain because blood collects under the nail.	1. Relieve pressure under the injured nail by using one of the following methods: • Use the eye end of a sewing needle or similar metal object. Hold the needle with pliers, and use a match or lighter to heat it until the metal is red hot. Press the glowing end of the needle against the nail so that it melts through. Little pressure is needed. The nail has no nerves, so this treatment is painless. Figure 8 OR • Using a rotary action, carefully drill through the nail with the sharp point of a knife. This method may be painful and takes more time. 2. Apply a dressing to absorb the draining blood and to protect the injured nail.

Amputations

What to Look For	What to Do
If a body part is amputated, immediate action is needed for reattachment. Amputated body parts that are left uncooled for more than 6 hours have little chance of survival.	1. Control the bleeding with direct pressure, and elevate the extremity. Treat for shock by laying the victim down, raising his or her legs, and keeping him or her covered. 2. Recover the amputated part, and take it with the victim.

(continued)

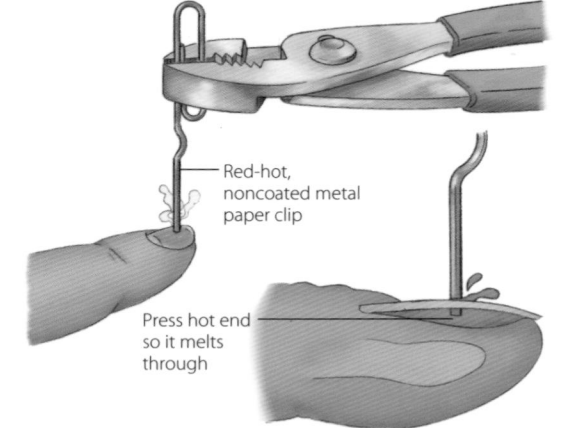

Red-hot,
noncoated metal
paper clip

Press hot end
so it melts
through

Figure 8

3. Care for the amputated part:
- If possible, rinse part with clean water;
  DO NOT scrub.
- Wrap part with a dry sterile gauze or clean
  cloth.
- Put the wrapped amputated part in a plastic bag or another waterproof container.
- Place bag or container with the wrapped
  part on a bed of ice. **DO NOT** bury it in ice.
4. Evacuate to medical help as soon as
   possible.

Animal Bites

Use the procedures found in Bleeding and Wound Care section. Animal bites have a high risk for infection; evacuate to medical help.

Blisters

These procedures are for friction blisters; do not apply to blisters related to poison ivy, burns, or frostbite.

What to Look For	What to Do
"Hot" spot (red, painful area caused by rubbing before becoming a blister)	1. In several pieces of moleskin or molefoam, cut an oval hole in middle the size of hot spot. If neither is available, tightly apply a piece of tape over the hot spot. Do not use an adhesive strip (e.g., band-aid). 2. Place the hole over the hot spot, and tape it in place. Apply several layers of the moleskin or molefoam to prevent rubbing against area.
Blister on foot is closed and not very painful (collection of fluid in a "bubble" under outer layer of skin caused by rubbing)	Either 1. Tape the blister tightly with tape OR 2. In several pieces of moleskin or molefoam, cut an oval hole in middle the size of the blister; place the hole over the blister, and tape it in place. Apply several layers of the moleskin or molefoam to prevent rubbing against area. *(continued)*

Bleeding and Wound Care » Blisters

Blister on the foot is open or is a very painful closed blister affecting walking	1. Clean area with soap and water or alcohol wipe. 2. Drain all of the fluid by making several small holes at base of blister with a sterilized needle. Press the fluid out. **DO NOT** remove the blister's roof unless it is torn. Figure 9 3. In several pieces of moleskin or molefoam, cut an oval hole in middle the size of the blister; stack the pieces on top of each other with the holes over the blister. Applying several layers of moleskin or molefoam prevents rubbing against area. 4. Apply antibiotic ointment in hole, and cover tightly with tape.

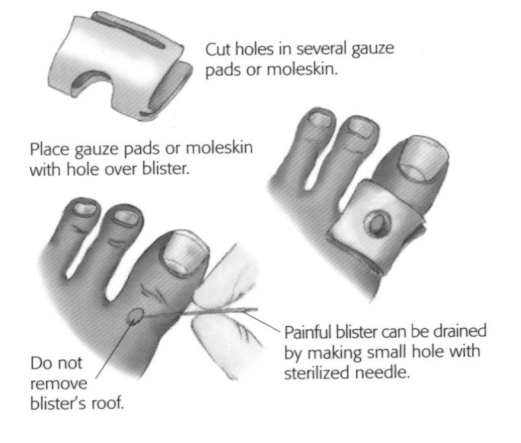

Cut holes in several gauze pads or moleskin.

Place gauze pads or moleskin with hole over blister.

Do not remove blister's roof.

Painful blister can be drained by making small hole with sterilized needle.

Figure 9

The blister's roof should be left on unless the blister is infected or is partially torn off. In these instances, use sterilized scissors to remove loose skin of the blister's roof up to the edge of the normal skin, and apply antibiotic ointment and sterile dressing.

Fishhook Removal

Do not try to remove a fishhook if it is near an eye, blood vessel, or nerve or if the victim is uncooperative. If the barb has not penetrated the skin, back the hook out, and treat the wound. If the hook's barb has entered the skin, use one of these methods:

1. Seek medical help if it is nearby, and have a physician remove it.
2. If you are in a remote area far from medical help, remove the hook using either the pliers method or the fishline method. Figure 10

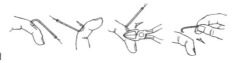

Pliers Method

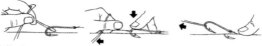

Fishline Method

Figure 10

Internal Bleeding

Internal bleeding is difficult to recognize. The victim may have received a hard blow or penetrating object to the chest or abdomen.

What to Look For

Pale, cool skin

Area hit may be discolored, tender, and swollen.

Fast breathing and pulse

Nausea and vomiting

Blood may be seen as

- Foaming red during coughing
- Red or brown during vomiting
- Black and tarry during bowel movement
- Red or smoky brown during urinating
- Oozing from the nose or ear or as a black eye(s)

What to Do

1. Check breathing.
2. Treat for shock—elevate legs and maintain body heat.
3. If unresponsive, place on side.
4. Seek medical help as soon as possible.

DO NOT give food or drink.

Bone, Joint, and Muscle Injuries

Broken Bones (Fractures)

What to Look For

It may be difficult to tell whether a bone is broken. When in doubt, treat the injury as a broken bone. Use "DOTS" in checking an injury:

- **D**eformity might be obvious. Compare the injured part with the uninjured part on the other side.
- **O**pen wound may have an underlying broken bone.
- **T**enderness and pain will be easily pointed out by the victim. A useful technique for detecting a fracture is to gently feel, touch, or press along the length of the bone; a victim's complaint about tenderness or pain is a reliable sign of a fracture.
- **S**welling happens rapidly after a fracture.

What to Do

1. Gently remove clothing covering injured area.
2. Check blood flow and nerves—for arm, feel for pulse at the wrist; for leg, feel for pulse behind ankle knob on inside). Ask the victim whether he or she feels you lightly squeezing the toes/fingers; ask the victim to wiggle the toes/fingers unless injured.
3. Use RICE procedures (discussed on the next page).
4. Give pain medication.
5. Stabilize in place by applying a splint.
6. Evacuate to medical help if victim cannot continue trip.

Evacuate as soon as possible for

- Open fractures (bleeding)
- No arm/leg pulse
- Broken thigh (femur) or pelvic bone

B

RICE Procedures

Use RICE for bone, joint, and muscle injuries. In addition to RICE, fractures and dislocations should be stabilized against movement with a splint. Figures 11 and 12

R = Rest. The victim should not use the injured part.

I = Ice. Cold should be applied as soon as possible for 20 to 30 minutes every 2 to 3 hours during the first 24 to 48 hours. Cold can be applied directly on the skin; however, a thin cloth or a paper towel placed over the skin prevents freezer burn.

C = Compression. Applying an elastic bandage reduces swelling. When not applying cold, apply compression (pressure). Place soft padding around the bones to compress the soft tissues to help reduce swelling.

E = Elevation. If possible, keep the injured part higher than the heart to decrease swelling and pain.

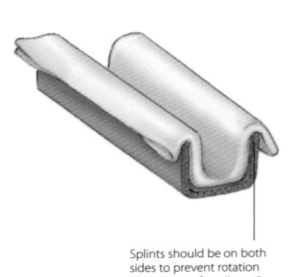

Splints should be on both sides to prevent rotation (shows use of cardboard).

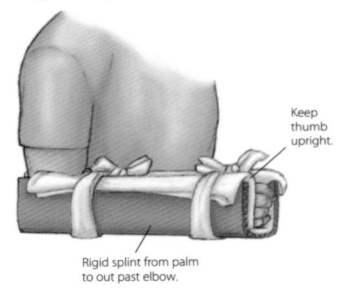

Keep thumb upright.

Rigid splint from palm to out past elbow.

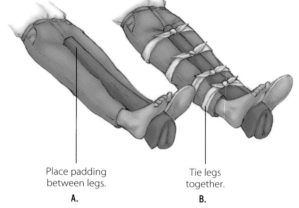

Place padding
between legs.

Tie legs
together.

A.

B.

Figure 12

Dislocated Joints: Shoulder, Kneecap, and Finger

A dislocation happens when a joint (e.g., shoulder, finger)
comes and stays apart. Joint deformity is obvious. Try to
reduce only anterior shoulders, kneecaps, and fingers.
Relocate as soon as possible because it is easier before
swelling and muscle spasms develop. *Do not* try to relocate
elbows, hips, ankles, wrists, or knees. It is difficult to distinguish from severe fracture, and methods are painful and
likely to cause injury.

What to Look For	What to Do

Anterior shoulder (95% of all shoulder dislocations)
· Victim cannot touch opposite shoulder with hand of injured arm
· Arm held away from body
· Extreme pain
	1. Check pulse at wrist, squeezing a finger for sensation, and wiggling fingers before and after.
	2. Methods (Use one of these)
	  · Simple hanging with 10 to 15 pounds of weight strapped to the wrist and lower arm (takes up to 60 minutes), Figure 13
	OR
	  · Traction and rotation. Slowly move arm into a "baseball throwing" position above the head (takes up to 10 minutes). Figure 14
	3. After reduction, stabilize shoulder with sling and swathe (binder).

Patella (kneecap) · The kneecap moved to the outside of knee joint (large bulge under skin) · Extreme pain	1. Bend hip toward chest and straighten leg. 2. You may need to push the kneecap back in place while straightening leg. 3. Splint with leg straight. The victim can usually walk on an injured leg.
Finger · Deformity · Unable to use · Compare with finger on other hand	1. Hold the end of the finger, and pull it in the direction it is pointing. Figure 15 2. While pulling, swing the finger back into normal alignment. 3. Splint with "buddy taping" with fingers slightly bent. Figure 16 Note: · Try reducing only once. · **DO NOT** try reducing joint at base of index finger or base of thumb (both require surgery).

Evacuate to medical help any dislocations that cannot be relocated (three named previously here) and those of the wrist, elbow, hip, knee, and ankle.

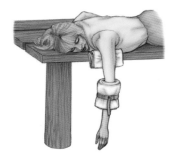

Figure 13

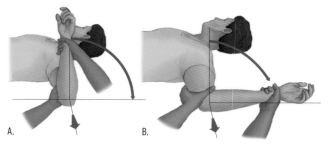

A.

B.

Figure 14

Bone, Joint, and Muscle Injuries » Dislocated Joints

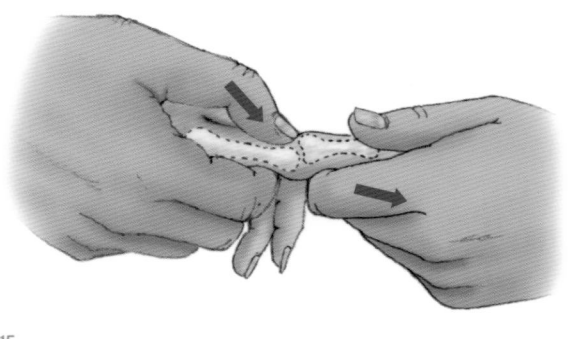

Figure 15

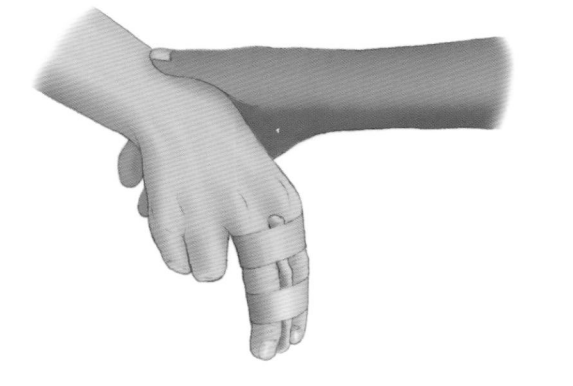

Figure 16

Ankle Injuries (Adapted from Ottawa Ankle Rules)

What to Look For	What to Do
If any pain or tenderness in ankle and 1. Bone tenderness/pain along the back edge or tip of the ankle knob bone (malleolus) when pushed on with the finger or thumb, and 2. Cannot bear weight and take four steps immediately after the injury and an hour later.	Suspect fractured ankle 1. Treat with RICE. 2. Stabilize against movement with a splint. 3. Evacuate to medical help.
If any pain or tenderness in ankle and 1. No bone tenderness/pain along back edge or tip of ankle knob bone (malleolus) when pushed on with finger or thumb, and 2. Can bear weight and take four steps immediately after the injury and an hour later.	Suspect sprained ankle 1. Treat with RICE. 2. No evacuation is needed. 3. **DO NOT** apply heat until 48 to 72 hours after injury. Figure 17

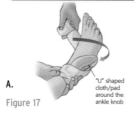

A.

"U" shaped cloth/pad around the ankle knob

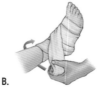

B.

Figure 17

Knee Injuries

What to Look For	What to Do
Use one of these procedures to check for a knee injury: Pittsburgh Knee Rules If a blunt trauma or a fall caused the injury, Plus one of the following: • Age < 12 years or > 50 years • Inability to walk four steps Another option is to use the Ottawa Knee Rules: • Age over 55 years • Tenderness at the patella (kneecap) • Tenderness at head of fibula (bony knob on outside of knee • Inability to flex knee to 90 degrees • Inability to bear weight and take four steps immediately after injury and an hour later	1. Treat with RICE. 2. Stabilize against movement with splint. 3. Evacuate to medical help.

Splinting Guidelines

All broken bones and dislocations should be stabilized before moving the victim. When in doubt, apply a splint. Any device can be used to stabilize a broken bone or dislocation. The device can be improvised (e.g., ski poles, canoe/kayak paddles, or pillow) or can be a commercial splint (e.g., a SAM Splint). A self-splint is one in which the injured body part is tied to an uninjured part (e.g., injured finger taped to adjacent finger, legs tied together, or arm tied to chest).

1. Cover all open wounds with a dry, sterile dressing.
2. Check blood flow and nerves—for an arm, feel for a pulse at the wrist; for a leg, feel for a pulse behind the ankle knob on the inside. Ask the victim whether he or she feels you lightly squeezing toes/fingers, and ask the victim to wiggle his or her toes/fingers unless injured.
3. Determine what to splint by using the "Rule of Thirds." Imagine each long bone as being divided into thirds. If the injury is located in the upper or lower third of a bone, assume that the nearest joint is injured. Therefore, the splint should extend to stabilize the bones above and below the joint. For a break of the middle third of a bone, stabilize the joints above and below the fracture. Any broken arm, in addition to being splinted, should be placed in an arm sling and binder (ties arm to chest).
4. If two first aid providers are present, one should support the injured part to minimize movement until splinting is finished.
5. If possible, place splint materials on both sides of the injured part, especially when two bones are involved (e.g., radius/ulna, tibia/fibula).
6. Apply splints firmly but not tightly enough to affect blood flow. Pad splints with clothing or other material for comfort.

Bone, Joint, and Muscle Injuries » Splinting Guidelines

7. Try to straighten a fracture in only remote locations and if one or both of the following exists: (1) an extremity is badly deformed and/or (2) no pulse can be felt. *Do not* move a suspected injured spine or replace a dislocation, *except* anterior shoulder, kneecap, and finger dislocations.

Muscle Injuries

What to Look For	What to Do
• Sudden muscle pain • A muscle, often the calf muscle of lower leg, that feels hard because of the muscle contraction • Often residual discomfort for a few hours	Suspect a muscle cramp (spasm): Try one or more of these to relax the muscle: 1. Have the victim gently stretch the affected muscle. 2. Press on the muscle. 3. Apply ice to the muscle. 4. For only a calf muscle cramp in the lower leg, have the victim pinch the upper lip hard (an acupressure technique). 5. Drink lightly salted cool water (one-fourth teaspoon salt in 1 quart of water) or commercial sports drink.
• A blow to a muscle • Swelling • Tender and painful • Black and blue mark appears hours later	Suspect a muscle bruise (contusion): Use the RICE procedures.

(continued)

- Happens during physical activity
- Sharp pain
- Very tender
- Cannot use injured part
- Stiffness and pain when muscle is used

Suspect muscle strain (pull):
Use the RICE procedures.

Evacuate these injuries as soon as possible (Wilderness Medical Society guidelines):

- A broken bone or dislocation with an open fracture
- No pulse felt in the extremity
- Suspected spinal cord injury
- Heavy blood loss
- Severe deformity affecting blood flow and/or sensation

Burns

1. Stop the burning! If clothing is on fire, have victim roll on the ground using the "stop, drop, and roll" method. Smother the flames with a blanket, or douse the victim with water. Remove clothing and all jewelry, especially rings, from the burn area. If it is a chemical burn, wash with large amounts of water. Dry chemicals should be brushed off before flushing with large amounts of water.

2. Check and monitor breathing if the victim breathed heated air or was in an explosion.

3. Determine the depth of the burn. This is difficult but helps determine what first aid to give.
4. Determine the size of the burn by using the "Rule of the Hand." The victim's hand (includes palm, fingers, and thumb) equals about 1% of victim's body surface area (BSA).
5. Determine which parts of the body are burned. Burns on the face, hands, feet, and genitals are more severe than burns on other body parts.

What to Look For	What to Do
First-degree burn (superficial)—redness, mild swelling, tenderness, and pain	1. Immerse the burned area in cold water, or apply a wet, cold cloth until pain free both in and out of the water (usually 10 to 45 minutes). If cold water is unavailable, use any cold liquid available.
	2. Give ibuprofen (for children, give acetaminophen).
	3. Have the victim drink as much water as possible without becoming nauseous.
	4. Keep burned arm or leg raised.
	5. After burn has been cooled, apply aloe vera gel or an inexpensive moisturizer. First-degree burns do not need to be covered.

(continued)

Small second-degree burn of less than 20% BSA (partial-thickness)—blisters, swelling, weeping of fluids, and severe pain	1. Follow same procedures (steps 1 through 4) as for a first-degree burn with these additions:
	2. After burn has been cooled, apply thin layer of antibacterial ointment (e.g., Bacitracin or Neosporin).
	3. Cover burn with a dry, nonsticking, sterile dressing or a clean cloth.
Large second-degree burn or more than 20% BSA (partial-thickness)	1. Follow steps 2–4 of first-degree burn care. Monitor for hypothermia (e.g., shivering, cold skin on unburned areas).
	2. Evacuate to medical help.
Third-degree burn (full-thickness)—dry, leathery, grayish, or charred	1. Cover burn with a dry, nonsticking, sterile dressing or clean cloth.
	2. Evacuate to medical help.

Evacuation

Most burns are minor and do not require medical help. Superficial and small partial-thickness burns rarely need medical help. Large partial-thickness and all full-thickness burns, burned airways, and circumferential burns (completely around body part) need medical help as soon as possible.

[Cardiac Arrest]

CPR

If you see a motionless person

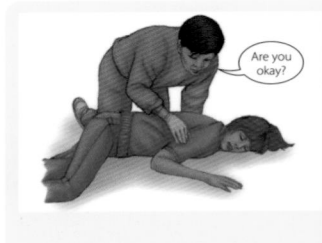

1. Check for responsiveness by tapping and shouting "Are you OK?" At the same time, check for breathing (i.e., chest movement). If there is no response (does not move or moan), place the victim onto his or her back, and if not breathing or has no normal breathing (i.e., only gasping), and depending upon the situation, either you or have someone else activate the emergency medical services.

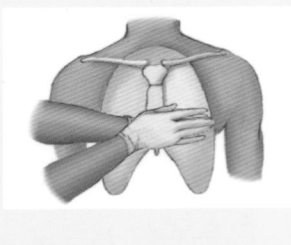

2. Give 30 chest compressions (push hard–at least 2 inches deep for adults, about 2 inches for children, at least 1.5 inches for infants; push fast–at least 100 per minute).

(continued)

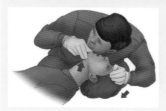

3. Open the airway (tilt head backward and lift chin upward).

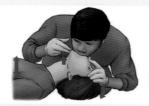

4. Pinch nose and give 2 breaths (1 second each) that make the chest rise.

(continued)

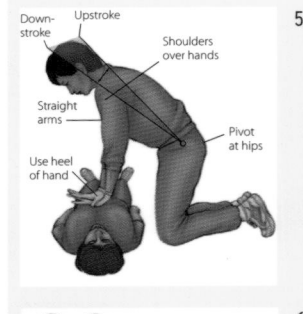

Down-
stroke   Upstroke

Shoulders
over hands

Straight
arms

Pivot
at hips

Use heel
of hand

5. Repeat cycles of 30 chest compressions and 2 breaths until you are exhausted, an AED is available, EMS personnel arrive, or 30 minutes has elapsed (except for hypothermic and cold water submersed victims; see page 59).

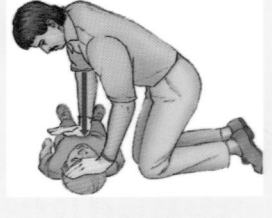

6. For children, use one or two hands (as for an adult) to depress the chest about 2 inches (one third) the depth of the chest. Use 30:2 compression to breathing ratio.

CPR in Remote Locations

After cardiac arrest, a victim's heart activity must be restored within a short time (most require medical help) for survival; thus, CPR is seldom successful in remote locations.

If . . .	Then . . .
If CPR is started in a remote location*	Continue CPR until • Victim recovers. • Rescuers are exhausted. • Rescuers are placed in danger. • The victim is turned over to higher trained personnel. • The victim does not respond to 30 minutes of resuscitation efforts.
If CPR is given for 30 minutes without success	Stop CPR. Exceptions when CPR can be given longer than 30 minutes: • Cold-water immersion of less than 1 hour • Avalanche burial • Hypothermia (for these victims, take 30 to 45 seconds to feel for a neck pulse before starting CPR) • Lightning strike

If any of these conditions are present:* **DO NOT** start CPR.

- Danger to rescuers
- Signs of death (e.g., rigor mortis or stiff, rigid muscles)
- Obvious lethal injury
- Documented do not resuscitate orders exist
- Victim has a rigid frozen chest

* Wilderness Medical Society guidelines

AED

Over 90% of cardiac arrest victims are in ventricular fibrillation (ineffective heart muscle contractions). Early defibrillation is the single most important factor in saving lives from sudden cardiac arrest. CPR alone usually will not reverse cardiac arrest, but it does buy time by allowing an AED to arrive and be applied. Most remote locations will not have an AED readily available.

Chest Injuries

Chest injuries can involve broken bones, penetrating injuries, and open or closed wounds.

What to Look For	What to Do
• Bleeding • Bruising • Deformity • Difficulty breathing • Impaled objects • "Sucking" sound during breathing	1. Monitor breathing and treat accordingly. 2. Impaled object: **DO NOT** remove; stabilize the object against movement. Seek medical help as soon as possible. 3. Sucking chest wound: seal the wound to prevent air from entering. Seek medical help as soon as possible. 4. Rib fracture: stabilize the ribs and chest with a coat, blanket, etc. The victim should cough, even though it is painful, a few times every hour to prevent pneumonia. Seek medical help. 5. **DO NOT** apply tight bandages around the chest.

[Chest Pain]

What to Look For	What to Do
Muscle or rib pain from physical activity or injury	Rest Aspirin or ibuprofen
Respiratory infection (pneumonia, bronchitis, pleuritis)–cough, fever, sore throat, and production of saliva	Needs antibiotic Seek medical help
Indigestion–belching, heartburn, nausea, and sour taste	Antacids
Angina pectoris–chest pain lasts less than 10 minutes	Rest If victim has physician-prescribed nitro-glycerin, help him or her take it (usually a small tablet).
Heart attack (see Heart Attack section)–the pain spreads to the shoulders, neck, or arms Lightheadedness, fainting, sweating, nausea, shortness of breath	1. Seek medical help as soon as possible. 2. Monitor breathing. 3. Place in half-sitting position. 4. If victim has physician-prescribed nitroglycerin, help him or her take one dose (may be small tablet, spray, or ointment). If it does not relieve the pain, seek immediate medical care. 5. If the victim is able to swallow and is not allergic to aspirin, help the victim take 1 adult aspirin (325 mg) or 2 to 4 chewable children's aspirins (81 mg each). Pulverize them or have the victim crunch them with his or her teeth before swallowing.

[Choking]

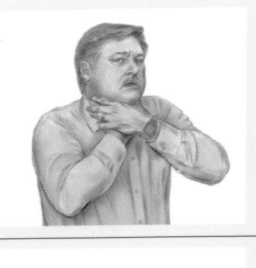

1. Check victim for choking. Ask "Are you choking? Can you speak to me?" A choking victim cannot breathe, talk, cry, or cough.

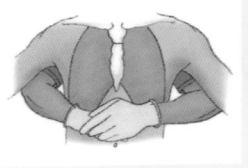

2. Give abdominal thrusts (Heimlich maneuver)
   · Position yourself behind victim
   · Place a fist against victim's abdomen, just above navel
   · Grasp fist with your other hand and press into victim's abdomen with quick inward and upward thrusts
   · Continue thrusts until object is removed or victim becomes unresponsive

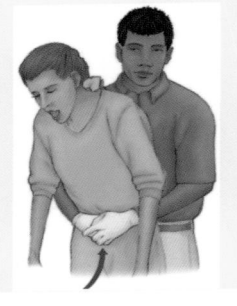

(continued)

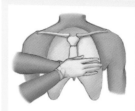

3. If victim becomes unresponsive and collapses onto ground
   - Begin CPR
   - After 30 compressions and each time you open the airway to give breaths, look for an object in the throat, and if seen, remove it.

C

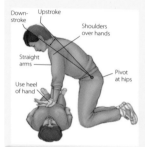

Down-stroke · Upstroke
Shoulders over hands
Straight arms
Pivot at hips
Use heel of hand

Choking

[Diabetic Emergencies]

Diabetes occurs when sugar in the blood builds up because of low insulin levels in the blood, thus not allowing the body's cells to get the energy that they need. People with diabetes take medication by mouth or injection, and carefully control what they eat (the source of energy) and their level of activity (use of energy).

A diabetic emergency results when too much insulin (insulin reaction or hypoglycemia) or too little insulin (diabetic coma or hyperglycemia) is in the blood. Figure 18

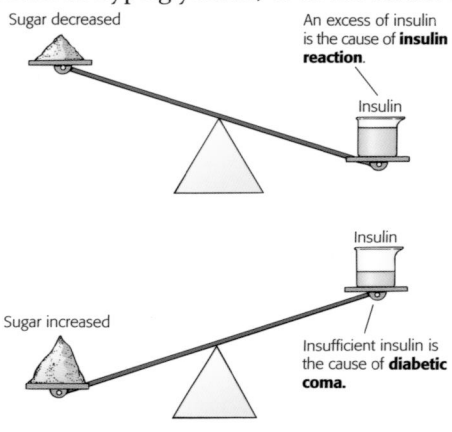

Sugar decreased

An excess of insulin is the cause of **insulin reaction**.

Insulin

Insulin

Sugar increased

Insufficient insulin is the cause of **diabetic coma.**

Figure 18

Low Blood Sugar (Insulin Reaction or Hypoglycemia)

What to Look For	What to Do
· Sudden onset · Staggering, poor coordination · Anger, bad temper · Pale color · Confusion, disorientation · Sudden hunger · Excessive sweating · Trembling · Eventual unconsciousness	If possible the diabetic should check his or her blood sugar. If it is not within a good range, or if the victim is a known diabetic with an altered mental status and is awake enough to swallow, he or she should follow the "Rule of 15s." 1. Give 15 grams of carbohydrate (e.g., 2 large teaspoons or lumps of sugar, or one-half can of regular soda, or 2 to 5 glucose tablets, or 1 tube of glucose gel). 2. Wait 15 minutes. 3. Have the victim check the blood sugar again and, if low, or if there is no improvement, eat 15 more grams of sugar. 4. Wait 15 minutes and check the blood sugar again and, if still low, or if there is still no improvement, seek immediate medical care.

D

High Blood Sugar (Diabetic Coma or Hyperglycemia)

What to Look For	What to Do
· Gradual onset · Drowsiness · Extreme thirst · Very frequent urination · Flushed skin · Vomiting · Fruity breath odor · Heavy breathing · Eventual unconsciousness	1. Give fluids. 2. Seek medical help. 3. If uncertain about whether the victim is in a diabetic coma or having an insulin reaction, give sugar using the "Rule of 15s."

[Eye Injuries]

Do not assume that an eye injury is minor. When in doubt, seek medical help as soon as possible.

E

What to Look For	What to Do
Blow to eye	1. Keep the victim on his or her back with the eyes closed. 2. Place an ice pack around eye for 15 minutes.
Loose object in eye	1. Try, in order, each step until one is effective: • Pull the upper eyelid down and over the lower lid. • Pull lower lid down, and look at inner surface while victim looks up. If object is seen, remove with wet gauze. • Lift the upper eyelid over a Q-tip. If an object is seen, remove it with wet gauze. 2. If successful, medical help is usually not needed.
Object stuck in eye	1. **DO NOT** remove the object. 2. If the object is long, place padding around object to stabilize and place paper cup or similar object over eye for protection. If the object is short, place a doughnut-shaped pad around the eye and hold in place with bandage wrapped around head. 3. Cover the uninjured eye with a bandage, but it may be necessary to leave a peephole to prevent anxiety.

(continued)

	4. Keep the victim flat on his or her back.
	5. Seek medical help as soon as possible.
Eyeball cut	1. **DO NOT** apply pressure to eye.
	2. Cover both eyes with gauze pads held by a bandage wrapped around head.
	3. Keep the victim's head raised.
	4. Seek medical help as soon as possible.
Chemical, smoke, or other irritant in eye	1. Hold the eye wide open; flush with warm water for 20 minutes.
	2. The eye(s) may need to be loosely bandaged.
	3. Seek medical help as soon as possible for chemical injury.
Light burns (from looking at sunlight or reflection off of snow or water): these burns may not be painful at first but become very painful hours later.	1. Cover both eyes with moist, cool cloths.
	2. Give pain medication (aspirin or ibuprofen) if needed.
	3. Seek medical advice.

E

Eye Injuries

[Female Health Problems]

Vaginitis

What to Look For	What to Do
· May have a white or yellowish discharge · Vaginal bleeding · Abdominal pain	1. Wash daily with plain water. 2. Wear loose-fitting underwear. 3. Wipe from front to back after a bowel movement or after urinating. 4. Seek medical help if there is lower abdominal pain and a fever or if foul-smelling vaginal discharge exists.

Urinary Tract Infection

What to Look For	What to Do
· Frequent urge to urinate · Burning while urinating · Blood in the urine	1. Drink more fluids—water is best. Avoid caffeine and alcohol. 2. Wear loose-fitting underwear. 3. Wash the area daily. 4. A hot bath may help relive pain and itching. 5. Wipe from front to back after a bowel movement or after urinating. 6. Seek medical help if symptoms last for 24 hours or if fever and chills occur.

For injury-related soft-tissue injuries, use direct pressure to control bleeding. Apply an ice pack to reduce swelling and pain. Apply a diaper-type bandage to hold dressings in place. Never place or pack dressings into the vagina. Seek medical help.

Noninjury vaginal bleeding can result form various causes, but the care is the same. Have the woman place a sanitary pad over the vaginal opening, and seek medical help.

Pregnancy Problems

- The "big three" warning signs of a serious problem: bleeding, abdominal cramps, and weakness. Seek medical help.
- Morning sickness, swollen ankles, and urinary tract infections are not usually dangerous, but seek medical advice.
- If a pregnant woman is "spotting," get her into bed immediately, as this could signal the onset of a miscarriage.

Frostbite

Frostbite happens only in below-freezing temperatures (< 32°F). It affects mainly the feet, hands, ears, and nose.

The most severe results are gangrene requiring surgical amputation. Check for hypothermia.

What to Look For	What to Do
Superficial frostbite · Skin color is white, waxy, or grayish yellow. · Affected part is cold and numb. · Might have a tingling, stinging, or aching sensation. · Skin surface feels stiff or crusty, and the underlying tissue feels soft when depressed gently. **Deep frostbite** · Affected part feels cold, hard, and solid and cannot be depressed—it feels like a piece of wood or frozen meat. · Affected part is pale, and the skin may appear waxy. · Painfully cold part suddenly stops hurting. · Blisters may appear after rewarming.	All frostbite injuries require the same first aid treatment: 1. Get the victim to a warm area. 2. Replace wet clothing or constricting items that could impair blood circulation (e.g., rings). 3. Do not rub or massage the area. 4. For deep frostbite, evacuate to medical help. 5. When more than 1 hour from a medical facility, place part in warm water (test by pouring some over the inside of your arm to test that it is warm, not hot). For the ear or face, it is best but may be difficult to apply warm moist cloths, changing them frequently. You may have to cover with warm hands. Give pain medication (preferably aspirin or ibuprofen). Rewarming may take 20 to 40 minutes when parts become soft. *Caution:* · **DO NOT** rub or massage part. · **DO NOT** apply ice or snow or cold water. · **DO NOT** rewarm with stove, vehicle's tailpipe exhaust, or over a fire. · **DO NOT** break blisters. · **DO NOT** allow the victim to smoke or drink alcohol.

(continued)

- **DO NOT** rewarm if there is any possibility of refreezing.
- **DO NOT** allow the thawed part to refreeze.

After thawing:

- Place a dry, sterile gauze between the toes and fingers to prevent sticking.
- Elevate the part to reduce pain and swelling.
- Give aspirin or ibuprofen for pain and inflammation. Do not give these to children.
- Apply a thin layer of aloe vera to the area.
- Seek medical help.

[Frostnip]

Frostnip is caused when water on the skin's surface freezes. It is difficult to tell the difference between frostnip and frostbite.

What to Look For	What to Do
• Skin appears red and sometimes swollen. • It is painful.	1. Gently warm the area against a warm body part (e.g., armpit, stomach, bare hands) or by blowing warm air on the area. 2. Do not rub area.

Frostnip 71

[Immersion Foot]

Immersion foot, also known as trench foot, occurs in non-freezing cold and wet conditions. This takes several days to occur.

What to Look For	What to Do
Feet are: • Cold, swollen, pale • Numb • Blotched with dark splotches	1. Dry and warm feet. 2. Give fluids to drink. 3. Give ibuprofen. 4. Evacuate to medical help.

Head Injuries

Suspect a spinal cord injury in head injured victims. Stabilize against movement until you have "cleared" the spinal cord (see the section on Spinal Cord Injury).

Scalp Wound

1. Control bleeding by pressing on wound. Replace any avulsed (torn) skin to its original position and apply pressure.
2. If you suspect a skull fracture, do not apply excessive pressure; this may push bone pieces into the brain. Press also on the edges of the wound.
3. Apply a dry, sterile dressing.
4. Keep the head and shoulders raised if no spinal cord injury is suspected.

Skull Fracture

What to Look For	What to Do
• Pain • Skull deformity • Bleeding from an ear or the nose • Leakage of clear, watery fluid from an ear or the nose	If you suspect a skull fracture: 1. Monitor breathing. 2. Control bleeding by pressing the edges of the wound and gently on the center of it. 3. Cover wounds with a sterile dressing. *(continued)*

- Discoloration around the eyes or behind ears appearing several hours after the injury
- Unequal-sized pupils of the eye
- Heavy scalp bleeding (skull and/or brain tissue may be exposed)
- Penetrating or impaled object

4. Stabilize the neck against movement unless you have "cleared" the spinal cord (see the section on Spinal Cord Injury).
5. Evacuate to medical help as soon as possible.
DO NOT clean the wound.
DO NOT remove an embedded object.
DO NOT stop blood or clear fluid that is draining from an ear or the nose.

H

Brain Injury (Concussion)

Injured brain tissue swells within the skull and produces the signs and symptoms described (American Academy of Neurology).

What to Look For	What to Do
<ul><li>Befuddled facial expression (vacant stare)</li><li>Slow to answer questions or follow instructions</li><li>Easily distracted</li><li>Walking in wrong direction; unaware of location</li><li>Slurred, incomprehensible speech</li><li>Stumbling, unable to walk a straight line</li></ul>	If you suspect a concussion: 1. Evacuate to medical help if unresponsive for any amount of time. 2. Suspect a spinal cord injury in head-injured victims. Stabilize against movement unless you have "cleared" the spinal cord (see the section on Spinal Cord Injury). 3. Monitor breathing. 4. Control scalp bleeding (see the section on Scalp Wound). *(continued)*

- Crying for no apparent reason
- Repeatedly asking same question that has already been answered
- Unable to give the months of the year in reverse order
- Unable to recall three objects 5 minutes later
- Unresponsive

5. Keep victim on his or her left side to help prevent inhaling vomit (vomiting often happens with head-injured victims).

Evacuation of Head-Injured Person (Wilderness Medical Society Guidelines)

No Evacuation Needed	Urgent Evacuation
· Minor injury · Alert and responsiveness · No bleeding disorder or medications which may increase bleeding risk	· Severe headache · Altered mental status · Skull fracture · Penetrating object · Persistent nausea and vomiting · Battles sign (skin discoloration behind and below ears) · Raccoon eyes (severe discoloration around eyes) · Loss of coordination · Loss of visual acuity · Appearance of clear fluid from nose or ears · Seizures · Relapse into unresponsiveness

[Heart Attack]

In a heart attack, the heart muscle tissue dies because its blood supply has been severely reduced or stopped.

What to Look For	What to Do
• Pressure, fullness, squeezing, or pain in the center of the chest lasting more than a few minutes • Pain spreading to the shoulders, neck, or arms • Chest discomfort with dizziness, fainting, sweating, nausea, or shortness of breath Heart attacks are difficult to determine. One third of all victims do not have chest pain.	1. Monitor breathing. 2. Help the victim to a comfortable position (half sitting). Stop activity. 3. Ask whether the victim takes medication for chest pain (nitroglycerin)—if so, help him or her take it. 4. Seek medical help as soon as possible. 5. If breathing stops, give CPR (see the Cardiac Arrest section).

[Heat-Related Illnesses]

Heat illnesses include a range of disorders. Some are common, but only heatstroke is life threatening. Untreated heatstroke results in death.

Heatstroke

Two Types of Heatstroke

There are two types of heatstroke: *classic* and *exertional*.

The common characteristics of *classic* heatstroke are as follows:

- Affects older people
- Affects those who are chronically ill and/or sedentary
- Affects those who are on medication
- Common during heat waves
- Victims are not sweating.

The common characteristics of *exertional* heatstroke are as follows:

- Affects young, healthy individuals who are not acclimatized to the heat.
- Usually occurs during strenuous activity.
- Sweating is prevalent in about 50% of the victims.

What to Look For	What to Do
• Extremely hot skin when touched—usually dry, but may be wet. • Altered mental status ranging from slight confusion, agitation, and disorientation to unresponsiveness.	Suspect heatstroke: Heat stoke is life threatening and must be treated as soon as possible. 1. Move the victim to a cool place. Monitor breathing. 2. Remove the clothing down to the victim's underwear. 3. Keep victim's head and shoulders slightly raised. *(continued)*

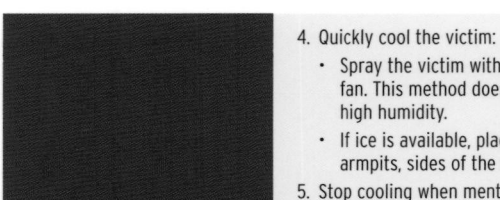

4. Quickly cool the victim:
   - Spray the victim with water and vigorously fan. This method does not work well in high humidity.
   - If ice is available, place ice packs into the armpits, sides of the neck, and groin.
5. Stop cooling when mental status improves or if shivering occurs.
6. Get medical help as soon as possible. Continue cooling during evacuation.

Heat Exhaustion

What to Look For

- Sweating
- Thirst
- Fatigue
- Flu-like symptoms (headache and nausea)
- Shortness of breath
- Rapid pulse

It differs from heatstroke by having (1) no altered mental status and (2) skin that is not hot, but clammy.

What to Do

Suspect heat exhaustion:

Uncontrolled heat exhaustion can evolve into heatstroke.

1. Move the victim to a cool place.
2. Have the victim remove excess clothing.
3. Have the victim drink cool fluids.
4. For more severe cases, give lightly salted cool water (dissolve one-fourth teaspoon salt in a quart of water) or commercial sports drink. Do not give salt tablets.
5. Raise the victim's legs 6 to 12 inches (keep the legs slightly bent).

(continued)

6. Cool the victim but not as aggressively as for heatstroke.
7. If no improvement seen within 30 minutes, seek medical help. Recovery may take up to 24 hours.

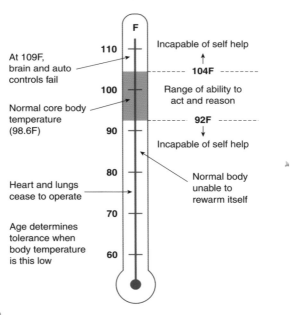

At 109F, brain and auto controls fail

Normal core body temperature (98.6F)

Heart and lungs cease to operate

Age determines tolerance when body temperature is this low

Incapable of self help
↑
---- 104F ----
Range of ability to act and reason
---- 92F ----
↓
Incapable of self help

Normal body unable to rewarm itself

Figure 19

Heat-Related Illnesses » Heat Exhaustion

Heat Cramps

What to Look For	What to Do
· Painful muscle spasms that happen suddenly · Affects the muscle in the back of the leg or abdomen · Occurs during or after physical exertion	Relief may take several hours. 1. Rest in a cool area. 2. Drink lightly salted cool water (dissolve one-fourth teaspoon salt in 1 quart of water) or a commercial sports drink. **DO NOT** give salt tablets. 3. For any cramped muscle, stretch it. For calf muscles in the lower leg, stretch the cramped calf muscle and/or try the acupressure method of pinching the upper lip just below the nose.

Heat Syncope

What to Look For	What to Do
· Victim is dizzy or faints · Seen immediately after strenuous physical activity in a hot environment	1. If the victim is unresponsive, check breathing. The person usually recovers quickly. 2. If the victim fell, check for injuries. 3. Have the victim rest and lie down in a cool area with legs raised. 4. Wet the skin by splashing water on the face. 5. If not nauseated and if fully alert and able to swallow, give lightly salted cool water (dissolve one-fourth teaspoon salt in 1 quart of water) or a commercial sports drink. **DO NOT** give salt tablets.

Heat Edema

What to Look For	What to Do
· The ankles and feet swell. · It occurs during first few days in a hot environment.	1. Wear support stockings. 2. Elevate legs.

Heat Rash (Prickly Heat)

What to Look For	What to Do
· Itchy rash on skin wet from sweating · Seen in humid regions after prolonged sweating	1. Dry and cool skin. 2. Limit heat exposure.

[Hypothermia]

Hypothermia happens when the body's temperature (98.6°F, 37°C) drops more than 2 degrees. Hypothermia does not require subfreezing temperatures. Severe hypothermia is life threatening. Check for possible frostbite.

For all hypothermic victims

   1. Stop the heat loss:
- Get the victim out of the cold.
- Handle the victim gently.

- Replace wet clothing with dry clothing.
- Add insulation (e.g., blankets, towels, pillows, and sleeping bags) beneath and around the victim. Cover the victim's head (50% to 80% of the body's heat loss is through the head).
- Cover the victim with a vapor barrier (e.g., tarp, plastic, and trash bags) to prevent heat loss. If unable to remove wet clothing, place a vapor barrier between clothing and insulation. For a dry victim, the vapor barrier can be placed outside of the insulation.
2. Keep the victim in a flat (horizontal) position.

Mild Hypothermia

What to Look For	What to Do
• Vigorous, uncontrollable shivering • Has the "umbles"—grumbles, mumbles, fumbles, stumbles • Has cool or cold skin on abdomen, chest, or back	1. Follow steps 1 and 2 above for all hypothermic victims. 2. Allow the victim to shiver—do not stop the shivering by adding heat. Shivering that generates heat will rewarm mildly hypothermic victims. 3. Give warm, sugary drinks, which can provide energy (calories) for the shivering to continue; they may also provide a psychologic boost. These drinks will not provide enough warmth to rewarm the victim.

(continued)

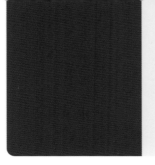

4. **DO NOT** give alcohol to drink—it dilates blood vessels, allowing more heat loss. Do not allow tobacco use.

5. Applying heat packs, hot water bottles, or body-to-body contact adds no advantage to rewarming those in mild hypothermia who are vigorously shivering. External rewarming increases skin temperature and stops shivering, which is undesirable.

6. If the victim is adequately rewarmed and has a normal mental status, evacuation to medical help is usually not needed.

Severe Hypothermia

What to Look For	What to Do
· Rigid and stiff muscles · No shivering · Skin feels ice cold and appears blue · Altered mental status · Slow pulse · Slow breathing · Victim may appear to be dead	1. Follow steps 1 and 2 above for all hypothermic victims. 2. Clothing on these victims should be cut off. 3. Monitor breathing, and give CPR if necessary. Check the pulse for 45 seconds before starting CPR. 4. Very gently evacuate to medical help for rewarming. Rewarming in a remote location is difficult and rarely effective. However, when the victim is far from medical help, the victim must be warmed by any available external heat source (e.g., body-to-body contact). *(continued)*

5. **DO NOT** start CPR if the victim:
   - Has been submerged in cold water for more than 1 hour
   - Has obvious fatal injuries
   - Is frozen (e.g., ice in airway)
   - Has a chest that is stiff or that cannot be compressed
   - Rescuers are exhausted or in danger

More cautions for all hypothermic care are as follows:
1. *Do not* give victim with altered mental status any warm drinks because this may cause choking and inhalation of the liquid.
2. *Do not* rub the extremities.
3. *Do not* place the victim in a shower or bath.

Lightning Injuries

Lightning is an electrical discharge that is associated with thunderstorms. The "Rule of 70s" about lightning strikes indicates that 70% occur in the afternoons, 70% during the summer months, 70% survive but may be injured or burned, 70% have an aftereffect, and 70% involve one victim. Lightning kills by stopping the heart and the breathing.

What to Look For

- Lightning strike seen or thunder heard in area. Rain may or may not be present.
- Minor burns on skin—the entrance and exit burn points common with electrical burns are rare with lightning. Types of burns
  - Punctate—small circular injuries resembling cigarette burns
  - Feathering or ferning—looks like feather or fern leaf
  - Linear burns
  - Ignited clothing and heated-metal burns
- May appear confused
- Muscle aches and tingling
- May be unresponsive

What to Do

Lightning victims are not "charged" and can be touched.

1. If more than one person has been struck, check first the breathing of those who are not moving and quiet.
2. Give CPR to those in cardiac arrest.
3. Check for spinal cord injury and treat.
4. If the victim is unresponsive but breathing, place him or her on his or her side.
5. Check for broken bones and dislocations and treat.
6. Check for burns and treat.
7. Evacuate to medical help even if responsive.

Marine-Animal Injuries

Injury Type	Marine Animal	What to Do
Bite, rip, or puncture	Sharks Barracudas Eels	1. Control bleeding. 2. Wash the wound with soap and water. 3. Flush the area with water under pressure. 4. Treat for shock. 5. Seek medical help.
Sting	Jellyfish Portuguese man-of-wars Anemone Fire coral	1. Apply vinegar to the sting area for at least 30 seconds. If vinegar is not available, use a baking soda paste. 2. Use hot water (110°F [43°C]) immersion or shower to reduce pain for at least 20 minutes. If hot water is not available, use hot dry packs. 3. Apply a coating of hydrocortisone (1%) several times daily.
Sting	Sea snake Octopus Cone shell	1. Apply a compression bandage on the entire bitten arm or leg. 2. Seek medical help.

(continued)

M

Injury Type	Marine Animal	What to Do
Puncture (by spine)	Stingray Scorpion fish Stonefish Starfish Catfish	1. Relieve pain by immersing part in hot water for 30 to 90 minutes or until pain subsides. Do not use water hot enough to cause a burn.
		2. Wash the wound with soap and water.
		3. Flush the area with water under pressure.
		4. Treat the wound.

[Motion Sickness]

What to Look For	What to Do
While traveling by car, truck, van, bus, train, ship, or airplane · Sweating · Dizziness · Pale skin · Nausea sometimes leading to vomiting	1. Stop activity if possible. 2. Take over-the-counter antinausea pills—known as Dramamine and Bonine. 3. Ingest ginger either as a solid or liquid or in capsules taken on an empty stomach. 4. Use thumb pressure or an acupressure wristband to apply pressure in the center of the wrist between the two forearm bones, two finger widths from the wrist crease. Press three to five times firmly for 1 minute, and then repeat on the other arm.

M

[Near-Drowning (Submersion)]

What to Look For

- Person floating on surface of water
- A swimmer who suddenly becomes motionless in the water
- A person who dives under the water and never reappears

What to Do

1. Rescue by using "reach-throw-row-go."
   - Reach = Reach with a long object (e.g., tree limb or rope) from shore.
   - Throw = Throw any object that floats (e.g., picnic jug or spare tire) or throw a rope and tow the victim to safety.
   - Row = Use a rowboat, raft, or canoe if available.
   - Go = If trained and skilled, swim to the person. Use a towel or board for him or her to hold onto. Do not let the person grab you. This can be a dangerous rescue.
2. Rescuers should provide CPR as soon as an unresponsive submersion victim is removed from the water. When rescuing a drowning victim of any age, a lone rescuer should give 5 cycles of CPR before leaving the victim to activate the EMS. Mouth-to-mouth breathing in the water may be helpful. Chest compressions are difficult to perform in water and may not be effective. Using abdominal thrusts is not necessary and can cause injury, vomiting, and delay of CPR.
3. Check for spinal cord injury for the victim who dove into water; protect the spine if a spinal injury is suspected (see the Spinal Cord Injury section).
4. Seek medical help as soon as possible even if victim feels "okay."

N

Nose Injuries

What to Look For	What to Do
Broken nose	1. If bleeding, care for the nosebleed. 2. Apply an ice pack for 15 minutes. 3. Medical help can be delayed. 4. **DO NOT** try to straighten a crooked nose.
Nosebleed	1. If nose was hit, suspect a fracture. 2. Sit the victim leaning slightly forward. 3. Pinch nostrils together for 5 minutes. 4. If bleeding has not stopped, gently sniff or blow the nose; pinch again for 5 minutes. 5. Try other methods in addition to nose pinching: apply an ice pack or apply decongestant spray in nostrils. 6. Medical help is not usually needed. If bleeding continues, seek medical help.
Foreign object (a problem mainly with children)	Try one or more of these methods: • Induce sneezing by sniffing pepper. • If an object is visible, pull the object out with tweezers. **DO NOT** push object deeper. • Gently blow nose while compressing the opposite nostril. • Seek medical help if the object cannot be removed.

N

[Plant-Related Problems]

Plant-Induced Dermatitis: Poison Ivy, Poison Oak, and Poison Sumac

Poison ivy can be found in every state except Hawaii and Alaska. Poison oak grows in some eastern states and along the West Coast. Poison sumac is found mainly in swampy areas on the East Coast, especially in the Southeast. Although these plants look different, the damage they do is similar. Figure 20

Poison ivy growing in one area may not look anything like poison ivy found halfway across the country, and poison oak of the East is very different from poison oak in the West. However, the dermatitis that these plants cause—and the treatment—is similar.

About 50% of the people exposed to these plants break out in a rash. The "poison" in these plants is the chemical urushiol, which is found in the sap. All parts of the plant— leaves, stems, roots, flowers, and berries—contain urushiol.

An allergic reaction may begin as early as 6 hours after exposure with a line of small blisters where the skin brushed against the plant, followed by redness, swelling, and larger blisters. The blister fluid does not contain the irritant. Usually, the onset of symptoms is 24 to 72 hours after exposure.

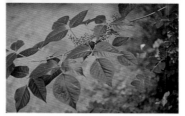

A. Poison ivy

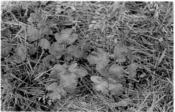

B. Poison oak

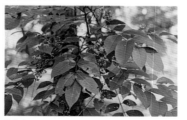

C. Poison sumac

Figure 20

Plant-Related Problems » Plant-Induced Dermatitis

As long as 2 weeks after the initial eruption, the rash may appear on other areas of the body. This can be explained by either (1) skin that erupts at a later time because it was exposed to less urushiol or (2) skin that is in different parts of the body differs in how it absorbs and reacts.

Poison ivy, oak, and sumac dermatitis are self-limiting conditions. Without any treatment, a mild case of any of these will often disappear in about 2 weeks. Usually the discomfort is too much, and the first aid procedures discussed here do not cure the condition but simply ease the suffering.

Over-the-counter hydrocortisone cream or ointment (1%) offers little benefit. Seek medical advice for severe cases.

Do not worry about giving the rash to others; it is not contagious. Animals can carry the sap on their fur. Smoke from burning plants can carry particles of the sap.

What to Look For	What to Do
Known contact within 5 minutes for sensitive people and up to 1 hour for moderately sensitive people	Cleanse skin with soap and lots of water or rubbing alcohol (isopropyl). Do not dap it on or use packaged alcohol wipes.
Mild: itching	Use any of these: · Oatmeal soaks (Aveeno) · Calamine lotion · Domeboro [Burow's solution (aluminum acetate)] · Baking soda paste (1 teaspoon of water mixed with 3 teaspoons of baking soda) *(continued)*

Moderate: itching and swelling	• Same as for mild signs and symptoms
	• Physician-prescribed cortisone ointment
Severe: itching, swelling, and blisters	• Same as for mild and moderate stages
	• Physician-prescribed oral cortisone
	• Evacuate to medical help if smoke from a burning plant is inhaled or if the reaction involves the face, eyes, genitals, or large areas of the body.

Cactus Spines

What to Look For	What to Do
Few cactus spines embedded in skin	Remove with tweezers
Many cactus spines embedded in skin	1. Coat the area with a thin layer of white woodworking glue or rubber cement.
	2. Allow it to dry for 30 minutes.
	3. Slowly roll up the dried glue from the edges.
	Adhesive tape or duct tape removes only some of the spines, even after many attempts.
	DO NOT use Super Glue.

P

Stinging Nettle

The stinging nettle plant has stinging hairs on its stem and leaves. Its effects are not an allergic response but are due to an irritant effect of the plant's sap.

What to Look For	What to Do
Rapid, intense burning sensation, itching	1. Wash the area with soap and water. 2. Apply a cold, wet pack. Could also use colloidal oatmeal, hydrocortisone cream (1%), or calamine lotion. 3. Take an antihistamine, if desired, following the package directions.

Swallowed (Ingested) Poisonous Plant

What to Look For	What to Do
· Abdominal pain and cramping · Nausea or vomiting · Diarrhea · Drowsiness	1. Determine: 　· The type of plant, if possible 　· How much was swallowed 　· When it was swallowed 2. For an alert, responsive victim, use a cell phone if available and if service is available to call the poison control center (the national number is 1-800-222-1222). Most poisonings can be treated through telephone instructions. *(continued)*

3. For an unresponsive victim, check breathing and treat accordingly. Evacuate to medical help as soon as possible.

4. Place the victim on his or her left side to delay poison's advance into the small intestine.

5. **DO NOT** try to induce vomiting.

6. Evacuate all mushroom-poisoned victims to medical help as soon as possible.

P

[Seizures]

Seizure results from a disturbance of the electrical activity in the brain causing uncontrollable muscle movements. Causes include epilepsy, head injury, brain tumor, stroke, heatstroke, poisoning—including alcohol or drugs, insulin reaction, or high fever.

What to Look For

- A sudden cry or scream
- A sudden loss of consciousness
- Rigid muscles followed by jerky movement with arching of the back (convulsions)
- Foaming at mouth
- Grinding of teeth
- Face and lips turn blue
- Eyes roll upward
- Loses bladder and bowel control

What to Do

1. Protect the victim from injury.
2. Loosen restrictive, tight clothing.
3. Roll onto side.
4. Seek medical help if any of these apply:
   - Nonepileptic victim
   - A seizure lasting more than 5 minutes
   - First-time seizure
   - Slow recovery
   - Pregnant victim
   - Injury related

S

[Shock]

Shock happens when the body's tissues do not get enough blood. Do not confuse this with an electric shock or "being shocked," as in scared or surprised. Shock is life threatening. Even if there are no signs of shock, you should still follow these procedures for injured victims.

What to Look For

- Altered mental status: anxiety and restlessness
- Pale, cold, and clammy skin, lips, and nail beds
- Nausea and vomiting
- Rapid breathing and pulse
- Unresponsiveness when shock is severe

What to Do

1. Treat injuries.
2. If responsive, lay the victim on his or her back and raise his or her legs 6 to 12 inches. If unresponsive, roll the victim on his or her side if no spinal cord injury is suspected.
3. Prevent body heat loss by putting blankets/coats under and over victim.
4. If not getting better, evacuate to medical help.

DO NOT raise the legs more than 12 inches.

DO NOT raise the legs of a victim with head injuries, stroke, chest injuries, breathing difficulty, or who is unresponsive.

DO NOT give anything to eat or drink.

S

Snake and Other Reptile Bites

For all snake and reptile bites:
- Get the victim and bystanders away from the snake or reptile because of the risk of a second bite.
- Keep the victim quiet.
- Gently wash the bite with soap and water.

Reptile	What to Look For	What to Do
Pit Vipers Figure 21 · Rattlesnakes · Copperheads · Cottonmouths · Water Moccasins Triangular, flat head, wider than the neck; vertical, elliptical pupils (cat's eye); and a heat-sensitive "pit" located between the eye and nostril · In about 25% of poisonous snakebites, there is no venom injected, only fang and tooth wounds (known as a "dry" bite).	· Severe burning pain at the bite site. · Two small puncture wounds (some may have only one). · Swelling within 10 to 15 minutes; can involve entire extremity. · Discoloration and blood-filled blisters possible in 6 to 10 hours. · Severe cases have nausea, vomiting, sweating, and weakness.	1. Identifying and killing the snake are not necessary. The same antivenin is used with bites from all North American pit vipers. 2. Evacuate to medical help. When possible, carry the victim. If alone and capable, walk slowly. *Caution:* **DO NOT** cut the victim's skin. **DO NOT** use mouth suction. **DO NOT** use any suction device. **DO NOT** apply cold/ice packs. **DO NOT** give alcohol. **DO NOT** apply electrical shock. Caution: A dead snake can still bite even if decapitated. *(continued)*

Coral snakes Small and very colorful, with a series of bright red, yellow, and black bands going all the way around its body. Every alternate band is yellow, and the snout is black. It is the most venomous snake in North America but rarely bites.	Few immediate signs. Absence of immediate symptoms is not evidence of a harmless bite. Several hours may pass before the onset of nausea, vomiting, sweating, tremors, drowsiness, slurred speech, blurred vision, swallowing difficulty, and breathing difficulty.	1. Apply mild pressure by wrapping several elastic bandages (e.g., Ace) over the bite site and entire extremity. 2. Do not cut or use suction. 3. Evacuate to medical help.
Nonpoisonous snakes Figure 22 If not sure, assume that the snake is poisonous.	Leaves a horseshoe shape of tooth marks on skin. There may be swelling and tenderness.	1. Treat the bite the same as a shallow wound. 2. Consult with a physician.
Venomous lizards such as the Gila monster (U.S. and Mexico) and the Mexican beaded lizard May firmly hang on during bite and chew venom into skin	• Puncture wounds—teeth may break off • Swelling and pain, often severe and burning • Sweating • Vomiting • Increased heart rate • Shortness of breath	1. Give pain medication. 2. Evacuate to medical help. 3. Use Pit Viper snake treatment section.

S

Snake and Other Reptile Bites

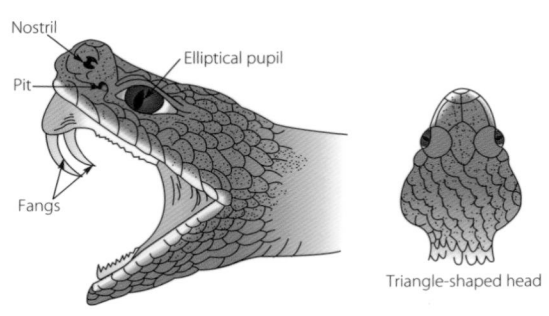

Pit Viper (venomous snake)
Figure 21

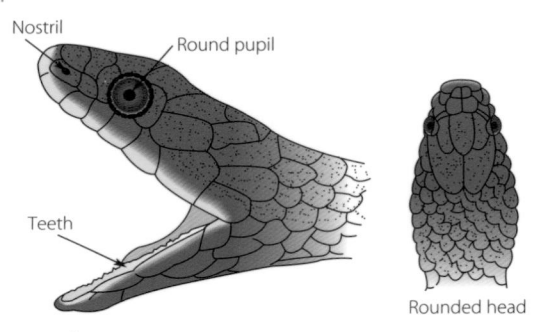

Nonpoisonous snake
Figure 22

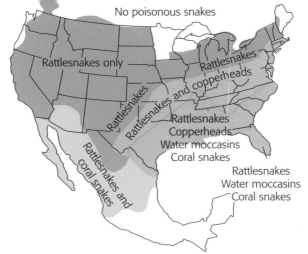

No poisonous snakes

Rattlesnakes only

Rattlesnakes and copperheads

Rattlesnakes

Rattlesnakes and copperheads

Rattlesnakes
Copperheads
Water moccasins
Coral snakes

Rattlesnakes and coral snakes

Rattlesnakes
Water moccasins
Coral snakes

Figure 23

[Spinal Cord Injury]

When a significant cause of injury (e.g., falls greater than three times the victim's height; a vehicle accident involving ejection, a roll-over, and high speeds; a head injury causing unresponsiveness; penetrations of the head, chest, or abdomen; diving into shallow water; or a head injury occurs, always suspect a spinal cord injury.

To stabilize a responsive person fully may not always be necessary because doing so is difficult, impractical, impossible, or dangerous to the victim.

A *reliable* victim does not need to be stabilized in one position if he or she meets the following criteria:

- Alert, knows name and where he or she is
- Not intoxicated by drugs/alcohol
- Calm, cooperative
- No painful, distracting injury

An *unreliable* victim is one or more of these:

- Unresponsive; altered mental status
- Intoxicated by drugs/alcohol
- Combative, confused
- Has a painful, distracting injury

What to Look For	What to Do
In a reliable victim	Suspect a spinal cord injury.
1. Complaints about back pain and leg numbness and tingling	1. Send for medical help. **DO NOT** attempt to evacuate the victim. Wait for trained personnel with proper equipment.
2. Tenderness/pain when you run fingers all the way down spine (if possible); press each bump of vertebrae and press on depressions on each side produced when you touch or push on the spine bones.	2. Leave the victim on the ground. Cover to prevent heat loss by log rolling the victim, keeping nose and navel pointing in the same direction, and place insulating materials under and over the victim.

(continued)

3. Fails these tests for sensation and movement (test all four extremities):
 	
 • Upper body:
 	
   a. Pinch several fingers and ask: Can you feel this? Where am I touching you?
 	
   b. Ask: Can you wiggle your fingers?
 	
   c. Have victim squeeze your hand.
 	
 • Lower body:
 	
   a. Pinch toes and ask: Can you feel this? Where am I touching you?
 	
   b. Ask: Can you wiggle your toes?
 	
   c. Have the victim push and pull a foot against your hand.
	3. Stabilize victim against movement. Kneeling and holding the victim's head with your hands quickly fatigues. Placing the victim's head between your knees is less tiring. Improvised cervical collars (e.g., SAM Splint, blanket) alone are inadequate. A method not requiring you to hold the victim constantly is improvising "sandbags" by placing dirt, sand, or rocks cushioned with clothing in stuff sacks or plastic bags and securely place them on both sides of the victim's head.

If these are *not* present in a reliable victim . . .	Suspect *no* spinal cord injury. Treat other injuries (e.g., wounds, bruises, fractures).
If the victim is unreliable and has a significant mechanism of injury (see above for examples) . . .	Assume that there is a spinal cord injury. Use the methods given above to stabilize the victim.

An injured victim who has an injury does not require spinal stabilization if he or she:

• is alert, not intoxicated, and has no distracting injuries
• has no complaints of neck pain or neurological symptoms (e.g., tingling, numbness)

- has no neck tenderness when felt, no loss of sensation when fingers and toes are pinched, and motion of the fingers and toes
- can rotate neck 45 degrees left and right when requested.

Stroke ("Brain Attack")

A stroke results when a blood vessel in the brain becomes plugged or ruptures so that part of the brain does not get the blood flow it needs.

What to Look For	What to Do
· Weakness, numbness, or paralysis of the face, an arm, or a leg on one side of the body	1. Monitor breathing.
· Blurred or decreased vision, especially in one eye	2. If responsive, place the victim in a half-sitting position. If he or she is unresponsive, place him or her in a recovery position.
· Problems speaking or understanding	3. Seek medical help as soon as possible.
· Dizziness or loss of balance	*Caution:*
· Sudden, severe, and unexplained headache	**DO NOT** give the victim anything to drink or eat.
· Suddenly falling or unsteadiness	
· Loss of bladder and bowel control	
· Unequal size of pupils	

S

Tooth Injuries

What to Look For	What to Do
• Toothache	1. Rinse mouth with warm water.
	2. Remove trapped food with dental floss.
	3. Use a cold pack on the outside of the cheek to reduce swelling.
	4. If available, use a cotton swab to paint the aching tooth with oil of cloves.
	5. **DO NOT** place aspirin on aching tooth or gum tissue.
	6. Give pain medication (e.g., aspirin, acetaminophen, and ibuprofen).
	7. Seek a dentist.
• Broken tooth	1. Rinse the mouth with warm water.
	2. Apply an ice pack on the face to decrease swelling.
	3. If a jaw fracture is suspected, stabilize the jaw by wrapping a bandage under the chin and over the top of the head.
	4. Seek a dentist as soon as possible.
• Knocked-out tooth	1. Rinse mouth and put rolled gauze pad in socket to control bleeding.
	2. Find the tooth, and handle by the crown, not the root.
	3. Rinse tooth with clean water; **DO NOT** scrub it.
	(continued)

T

4. Replace tooth into socket. Push down on tooth so the top is even with adjacent teeth. Biting down gently on gauze placed between the teeth is helpful.

5. If replacing tooth is not possible, transport tooth in saliva (< 1 hour) with victim to dentist.

[Wild Animal Attacks]

Human injuries by wild animals are rare, yet people often have fear and apprehension about venturing into wild areas. Much of these reactions come from myths, ignorance, exaggeration, and sensationalism. Most wild animals try to avoid people, and when attacks do occur they often result in only minor injuries. Traveling in a group is safer than being alone. In North America the wild animals that are most commonly reported as interacting with people include bears, bison, moose, cougars, coyotes, and alligators. Not all injuries are bites. Severe injuries result from victims being thrown in the air, gored by antler, butted, or trampled on the ground. Injures include puncture wounds, bites, lacerations, bruises, fractures, rupture of internal organs, and evisceration. The majority of wild animal attacks occur outside of the United States (for "What to Do," see the Bleeding and Wound Management section). Evacuate to medical help as soon as possible.

W

Prevention

Prevention: Altitude Illness

1. *Do not* rush to your destination. At higher elevations, start slowly and avoid overexertion. Those not accustomed to high altitudes should not ascend rapidly to sleeping altitudes greater than 10,000 feet and should spend 2 to 3 nights at 8,000 to 10,000 feet before going higher, with 1 extra night for every 2,000 to 3,000 feet. You can climb or ski higher during the day and return to a lower elevation at night ("climb or ski high, sleep low").
2. Drink lots of water (see the Prevention: Dehydration section for information).
3. Eat a high-carbohydrate diet because the appetite is often suppressed; also, food may be less available, and energy needs are greater.
4. *Do not* take sleeping pills because they cause shallow breathing while sleeping.
5. *Do not* smoke because it increases carbon monoxide blood levels, lessening the body's ability to use oxygen.
6. Ask your physician about the possible use of the medication acetazolamide (Diamox), which can prevent symptoms of acute mountain illness.

Prevention: Avalanche Burial

An avalanche is a mass of snow that slides down a mountainside.

1. Before going into potential avalanche country, call the nearest avalanche hotline to get the latest information about mountain weather, snow, and avalanche conditions.

2. Only one person at a time should go onto a slope that looks risky. Other people should serve as spotters from a safe location.

3. Avoid the center of open slopes. Cross an open slope at the very top or bottom.

4. Stay on shallow slopes. Avalanches most often start on slopes that are 30 to 45 degrees. Areas where avalanches occur year after year should be avoided. Figure 24

Avalanche Slope Angle

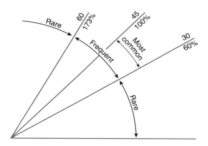

Figure 24

5. Do not travel alone.
6. If caught in an avalanche:
   - Try to escape to the side of the avalanche. Do not try to outrun by going downhill on skis or snowmobile.
   - Try to grab a tree.
   - Try to swim with the moving snow, similar to body surfing in the ocean.
   - Try to get away from a snowmobile, and get rid of ski poles.
   - Try to burst through the surface before the avalanche stops and clear a breathing space over your mouth.

Prevention: Bear Attack

Bear attacks rarely happen. Most encounters end without injury.

1. Avoid areas where high bear activity has been recently reported.
2. Try to avoid surprising a bear by making noise; hike with a group.
3. Hike during daylight hours.
4. Never approach a bear.
5. Recognize the signs of a bear (e.g., footprints, droppings, and scratches against trees with hair left).

6. Avoid using highly odorous foods that may attract a bear.

7. Properly store your food and garbage at all times except when they are being transported, prepared, or used. Store all food in vehicles or high in a tree—away from the sleeping area. Deposit garbage in refuse container or store as you would food. Do not bury it.

8. Never feed bears.

9. If a bear charges you:
   - *Do not* run—you cannot outrun a bear; try to remain calm.
   - *Do not* climb a tree—black bears and young grizzlies can climb trees.
   - *Do not* make quick movements; talk to the bear in a normal, monotone voice.
   - *Do not* stare directly at the bear.
   - If you have pepper spray, prepare to use it.
   - If the bear makes a bluff charge, stand quietly in a nonaggressive stance. In most cases, the bear stops the charge without making contact or causing injury. At this point, leave the area in the opposite direction from the bear.
   - For a black bear without cubs, try to chase it off with mild aggression—yell, shout, blow a whistle, throw rocks, and bang pots. If the bear does not leave, back away and leave the area.

10. During an attack:
   - Keep a backpack on for protection.
   - If you have pepper spray (oil-based capsaicin), spray the bear's eyes when the bear gets within about 20 feet. Continue spraying until the bear stops its charge; the spray lasts from four to nine seconds.
   - If it is a black bear, fight back by yelling, throwing rocks or sticks or whatever is available, and hitting and gouging the bear with your feet, fists, sticks, rocks, shovels—anything you have. Figure 25
   - If it is a brown bear (grizzly, Kodiak), play dead. Drop to the ground as the bear touches you—not before—and curl into a ball, covering your neck and head with your hands and arms. *Do not* struggle or fight back, and keep quiet. If the bear swats at you, roll with it. Stay face down and *do not* look around, and *do not* get up until you are sure it is gone.

If any bear preys on you, try to get away, shout for help, fight for your life, and defend yourself with anything available.

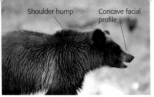

A. Grizzly bear

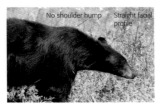

B. Black bear

Figure 25

[Prevention: Blisters]

1. Buy shoes or boots with adequate room in the toe box and with a good fit in the heel. They should be a size to a size and half larger than your dress shoes.
2. Wear socks made of CoolMax or polypropylene next to the foot to wick moisture away from the foot. Corn starch, talcum powder, baby powder, and antiperspirant also help to keep feet dry.

3. Wear a second pair of socks to prevent friction on the foot itself. Do not wear cotton socks.

4. Coat areas of foot prone to blister with a blister-chafing prevention agent such as petroleum jelly or AD ointment.

5. For areas that are already raw or very prone to blister, cover with moleskin.

6. Stop whenever you feel a hot spot developing, and cover the area with moleskin, molefoam, athletic tape, or duct tape.

7. Change wet socks and into dry ones when possible.

Prevention: Cold-Related Emergencies (Colorado Mountain Club)

Seek and create shelter from cold, wind, snow, and rain:

1. If possible, retreat to timbered areas for shelter construction and fire.

2. Use natural shelters: the windless side of ridges, rock croppings, slope depressions, snow blocks, a snow hole at the base of standing trees, dense stands of trees, or downed trees.

3. Improvise a windbreak or shelter from stacked rocks or snow blocks, tree trunks, limbs, and bark slabs and evergreen boughs, or dig a snow cave or snow trench with a cover. Figure 26

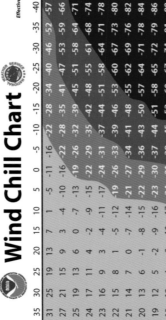

Figure 26

Conserve, Share, and Create Warmth

1. Conserve body heat by putting on extra clothing. Replace damp clothing and socks. Loosen boot laces to increase circulation. Use an Ensolite pad or evergreen boughs to insulate the body from the ground. Place hands in your armpits or crotch.

2. Share body heat. Sit or lie front to back or back to back. Warm the hands and feet of the injured person or companion.

3. Create body heat. Nibble high-energy goods—candy, nuts, or granola bar. Sip water that is kept warm with body heat. Use a solid fuel hand warmer, igniting both ends of fuel stick (good for 4 hours of heat). Do isometric exercises to stir the body's circulation system.

4. Build a fire. Find dry wood—dead lower branches and bark from underside of trees. Look under downed trees and inside of dead logs for dry kindling. Wet wood will burn as it dries in a strong fire. Select a sheltered area, protected from strong winds, as the site for an emergency campfire. Under snow conditions, build a fire base first, with large 4-inch diameter or larger pieces of wood (use wire saw). Put fire starter on the base. Surround the fire starter with branches to hold kindling above the fire starter, and then place a hatch work of kindling and slightly larger wood on the branches. Light the fire starter, and blow lightly to

help its flame ignite kindling. Add progressively larger wood to the flame area.

5. *Do not* drink alcoholic beverages because they:
   - cause frequent urination resulting in dehydration
   - dilate the skin's blood vessels, allowing more heat loss

6. Prevent heat loss. Remember that the body loses heat by respiration, evaporation, conduction, radiation, and convection.
   - To prevent loss by respiration, cover the mouth and nose with loosely woven wool or fleece.
   - To reduce evaporation through excessive perspiration, wear clothes that breathe and are in layers.
   - To avoid loss by conduction, use the Ensolite pad and/or other cover between the body and a cold, wet surface. This insulation is particularly important if you are already wet.
   - To prevent loss by radiation, keep the head, hands, and feet covered.
   - To prevent loss by convection, protect the body from the wind.

Clothing

1. Wear a base or first layer of clothing made of polypropylene.
2. Wear an insulating or second layer consisting of shirt and pants made of wool, fleece, or down.

3. Wear outer layers made of a windproof and water-resistant jacket that is worn loosely.
4. *Do not* wear cotton, as it does not wick sweat and will cool you rapidly if it gets wet.
5. Wear a stocking cap to insulate the head and retain heat. It should be large enough to cover the ears.
6. Wear a thin pair of gloves (or liners) inside a heavy wool or fleece mitten inside a Gore-Tex shell.
7. Remove layers as you warm up to prevent excessive sweating.
8. Keep clothing dry from rain, snow, and sweat.
9. *Do not* wear tight shoes/boots or too many socks or tie them so tight that they restrict blood flow.

[Prevention: Dehydration]

The body operates more efficiently when it is well hydrated. Dehydration causes more problems with most of the conditions described in this field guide, making them more severe and difficult to deal with.

How Much Fluid to Drink?

The Institute of Medicine recommends 13 cups of water and other beverages; for women, about 9 cups. Special attention should occur when:

- You are physically active.
- Your temperature exceeds 80° F.

- There is low humidity.
- You are at elevations above 5,000 feet.

How can you tell whether you are drinking enough?

- Check your urine—scanty, strong-smelling, dark urine signals that you need to drink more.
- Color of urine can be affected by medications, vitamins, and diet.
- If you feel thirsty, you are about 1% to 2% dehydrated.

Can you drink too much water?

- If you overhydrate (drink too much), sodium concentrations can drop (hyponatremia), allowing water to leak into brain cells, causing headache, confusion, personality changes, and even seizures, coma, or death.
- During physical activity, stay within the range of about 1.5 to 3.0 cups per hour.

Can commercial sports drinks be used?

- During strenuous physical activity in hot environments lasting over 1 hour, commercial sport drinks may be used.
- *Do not* take salt tablets.
- Snack foods can be useful if they contain some sodium.

Prevention: Drowning

1. Acquire swimming, rescue, and life-saving skills.
2. Learn how to row a boat and paddle a raft and canoe safely.

3. Children should be supervised by an adult when they are near or in the water.
4. Everyone on a boat, canoe, or raft should have a U.S. Coast Guard-approved life jacket on that will support the person with the head above water, even if the person is unresponsive.

[Prevention: Heat Stress]

1. Keep as cool as possible.
   - Avoid direct sunlight when possible.
   - Wipe cool water on exposed areas of the skin and/or place wet towels or ice bags on the body and/or dampen clothing.
   - Take cool baths or showers.
   - Dip clothing into water periodically, if possible.
2. Wear lightweight, porous, loose-fitting clothing that reflects heat, facilitates evaporative heat loss, and allows air to circulate around your body.
3. Wear a broad-brimmed hat.
4. Apply sunscreen.
5. Avoid, when possible, strenuous physical activity, particularly in the sun and during the hottest part of the day.

Heat Index

| Relative Humidity, % | Actual Thermometer Reading (°F) | | | | | | | | | | |
| | 70 | 75 | 80 | 85 | 90 | 95 | 100 | 105 | 110 | 115 | 120 |
	Apparent Temperature (°F)										
0	64	69	73	78	83	87	91	95	99	103	107
10	65	70	75	80	85	90	95	100	105	111	116
20	66	72	77	82	87	93	99	105	112	120	130
30	67	73	78	84	90	96	104	113	123	135	148
40	68	74	79	86	93	101	110	123	137	151	
50	69	75	81	88	96	107	120	135	150		
60	70	76	82	90	100	114	132	149			
70	70	77	85	93	106	124	144				
80	71	78	86	97	113	136					
90	71	79	88	102	122						
100	72	80	91	108							

Above 130° F = heatstroke imminent
105°F to 130°F = heat exhaustion and heat cramps likely; heatstroke with long exposure and activity
90°F to 105°F = heat exhaustion and heat cramps with long exposure and activity
80°F to 90°F = fatigue during exposure and activity

Source: National Weather Service

6. Drink enough water. Thirst indicates that you may be 1% to 2% dehydrated. Urine should be clear and occur an average of five times daily. Drink 1 cup (8 oz.) every half hour during strenuous activity. (See Prevention—Dehydration section.)
7. *Do not* use salt tablets.
8. *Do not* drink alcoholic beverages (e.g., beer and wine).
9. Rest frequently in shade.
10. Adapt to the heat (acclimate) by exercising in the heat 60 to 90 minutes each day for 1 to 2 weeks.

Prevention: Insect Stings (Bees, Wasps, Hornets, and Yellow Jackets)

1. *Do not* walk barefoot.
2. Insect repellents do not work against stinging insects.
3. *Do not* swat or flail at a flying insect. If need be, gently brush it aside or patiently wait for it to leave.
4. *Do not* drink from open beverage cans. Attracted by the sweet beverage, stinging insects will crawl inside a can.
5. When eating outdoors, try to keep food covered at all times.
6. *Do not* wear sweet-smelling perfumes, hair sprays, colognes, or deodorants.

7. *Do not* wear bright colored clothing with flowery patterns, which attracts flying insects.
8. Wear long pants and long-sleeved shirts.

Prevention: Lightning Strike (National Lightning Safety Institute)

If you can see lightning and/or hear thunder, you are already in danger. Louder or more frequent thunder indicates that lightning activity is approaching, increasing the risk for lightning injury or death. Estimate the distance in miles you are from a lightning flash by counting in seconds the time from when the flash is seen until the time the thunder is heard, and divide that number by five.

Use the "30-30 rule"—when the time between seeing the flash (lightning) and hearing the bang (thunder) is less than 30 seconds (this is the first "30") or 6 miles, you should be in or seek a safer location. Outdoor activities should not be resumed until at least 30 minutes (second "30") after the last lighting is seen or thunder heard.

1. When outdoors during a lightning/thunder storm:
   - Avoid water (lakes, rivers, etc.).
   - Avoid high ground.
   - Avoid open spaces where you are one of the tallest objects.

- Avoid a single tree or other high object (e.g., rock and bush).
- Avoid all metal objects including fences, machinery, etc.
- Avoid small, isolated sheds, rain shelters, etc.

When possible, find shelter in a substantial building or in a fully enclosed metal vehicle such as a car or truck with the windows completely shut. Do not touch any of the vehicle's inside metal.

2. If lightning is striking nearby when you are outside:
   - Squat like a baseball catcher. Put your feet together. Place your hands over ears to minimize hearing damage from thunder. Do not lie flat on the ground.
   - A group of people should spread out and stay a minimum of 15 feet apart.
3. If caught outdoors and no shelter is nearby:
   - Find a low spot away from trees, fences, and poles.
   - If you are in a forest, take shelter under the shorter trees or low brush.
   - If you feel your skin tingle or hair stand on end, squat down like a baseball catcher.
4. If boating, try to get to shore as soon as possible.
5. When indoors:
   - Stay away from fireplaces and metal pipes, and open doors and windows.

- Do not use a plugged in telephone (cell phones are safe).
- Turn off, unplug, and stay away from appliances, power tools, TV sets, etc.

Prevention: Mosquito Bites

1. Wear protective clothing during dawn and dusk or in areas where mosquitoes are active: long pants, long-sleeved shirt, and socks and shoes. For some areas, consider mosquito netting draped over a hat to protect face and neck.
2. Apply insect repellent containing DEET on exposed skin. Do not use a product with more than 30% DEET on people older than 5 years. Do not exceed 10% DEET for those under 5 years old.
3. Apply permethrin (kills, is not a repellent) only on clothing and not the skin.
4. Limit outdoor activities or take precautions given above at dawn and dusk.

Prevention: Mountain Lion Attack

1. Travel with others.
2. Keep small children close.

3. Obey warning signs or notices of mountain lion activity.
4. If you encounter a mountain lion:
   - *Do not* approach it; slowly back away. *Do not* turn your back to it.
   - *Do not* run—it may trigger an attack.
   - *Do not* make direct eye contact.
   - Appear larger than you are—raise arms above your head and make steady waving motions.
   - Yell or shout.
   - If small children are with you, pick them up.
   - If attacked, use anything as a weapon—a rock, branch, knife, or other hard object. If you have it, use pepper spray (capsaicin-based).

Prevention: Poisonous Plant Dermatitis

1. Learn to recognize and avoid the plants (poison ivy, poison oak, and poison sumac).
2. Wear long pants and long-sleeve shirts as protective clothing.
3. Apply an appropriate over-the-counter barrier cream (e.g., Ivy Block, Work Shield). Replenish the barrier protection every 4 to 6 hours when possible.
4. Wash or dispose of all contaminated clothing.

Prevention: Snakebite

1. *Do not* handle venomous snakes—keep away but do not kill them.
2. *Do not* hike and camp in snake-infested areas; avoid caves, rock crevices, dens, stonewalls, and wood piles.
3. Watch where you sit and step; *do not* sit on or step over logs until closely checked. *Do not* reach into holes or hidden ledges.
4. Wear protective gear such as boots, long pants, and long-sleeved shirts.
5. *Do not* handle a dead venomous snake. The reflex action of the jaws can still inflict a bite 20 minutes or more after the snake is dead, even if decapitated.
6. *Do not* surprise or corner a snake. Use a walking stick to prod uncleared ground, and make noise so that a snake can sense you coming.
7. Check bedding, clothing, and shoes/boots before use.

Prevention: Tick Bite

Ticks like to rest on low-lying brush and "catch a ride" on a passing animal or person. Areas with a high risk of ticks are wooded areas, low-growing grassland, and the seashore.

Ways to reduce chances of getting a tick bite include the following:

1. Avoid tick-infested areas, when possible—avoid short-cuts through heavily wooded, tick-infested areas.
2. In tick-infested areas stay in the center of paths, avoid sitting on the ground, and check clothing.
3. Dress properly.
   - Wear light-colored clothing so that ticks can be seen more easily and removed before becoming attached.
   - Wear a long-sleeved shirt that fits tightly at the wrists and neck, and tuck your shirt into your pants.
   - Wear long pants; tuck pant legs into boots or socks, or use masking or duct tape to secure pant legs tightly to socks, shoes, or boots.
4. After coming indoors, shower or bathe. Look and feel your entire body for ticks, especially in areas that have hair or where clothing was tight. Have a companion or use a mirror to check the scalp, behind and in the ears, neck, back, and behind the knees.
5. Use chemicals:
   - Apply insect repellents containing EPA-approved DEET to clothes and exposed skin. Avoid high-concentration products (more than 30% DEET) to the skin. Do not inhale or ingest DEET-containing

products or get them in your eyes. Do not use products with more than 10% DEET on children under 5 years of age.

- Apply 0.5% permethrin (kills ticks on contact) only to clothing and not the skin. Apply according to label instructions. Applications to shoes, socks, cuffs and pant legs are most effective against ticks.

Prevention: Waterborne Diseases

There are three main ways of making water safe to drink: boiling, chemicals, and special filters. Before using any of these methods, cloudy or dirty water should first be filtered through a clean cloth or through one of the commercial filters that does this (not all do), allowing the sediment to settle.

Boiling

Bringing water to a full boil for 1 full minute at any altitude makes the water safe to drink.

Chemicals

Both iodine and chlorine are inexpensive and are available in tablet or liquid. Iodine is preferred but should *not* be used if these conditions exist:

- Thyroid disease
- Iodine allergy
- Pregnancy

In all other persons it should not be used for more than a few months.

Iodine does not kill *Cryptosporidium*. Chemicals take longer to work in cold water and require larger amounts for cloudy or dirty water. Follow the manufacturer's directions concerning the amount administered.

Special Filters

Filters are expensive but simple to use. Filters are *not* a reliable method of removing viruses.

NOTES:

NOTES:

NOTES: